Praise for

FREE YOUR **FASCIA**

"If you want to feel better, look better, be happier, and feel younger, this book is a must-read. In it, Dr. Fenster tells you why freeing your fascia is vital to leading an energetic, pain-free life—and he tells you, step by step, just how to do it."

— **Dr. Fabrizio Mancini**, America's #1 healthy-living media expert, world-renowned chiropractor, international best-selling author and speaker, business consultant, and president emeritus of Parker University

*"As a master's certified practitioner of Active Release Techniques, it is refreshing to read a book that understands the importance of fascia. This is an area of soft-tissue rehabilitation that cannot be overlooked in the treatment of pain syndromes. **Dr. Daniel Fenster** has done an outstanding job. Kudos!"*

— **Christopher Anselmi**, DC, ART

*"In this exciting and informative book, **Dr. Daniel Fenster** introduces you to one of the most important and mysterious organs in your body— the fascia. He teaches you how to optimize your fascia, improving your flexibility, mobility, and ultimately your overall health."*

— **Dana Cohen**, M.D.

*"Having known **Dr. Daniel Fenster** professionally for over 30 years and seen the success of his work, this book is the grand culmination of those years. His comprehensive approach to understanding and treating fascia is second to none."*

— **Oz Garcia**, nutritionist

"Fascia is a very important subject in exercise, and this book examines fascia thoroughly."

— **Harley Pasternak**, nutrition expert and celebrity trainer

FREE YOUR
YOUR
FASCIA

Hay House Titles of Related Interest

FREE
YOUR
FASCIA

RELIEVE Pain,

BOOST Your Energy,

EASE Anxiety and Depression,

LOWER Blood Pressure, and

MELT YEARS Off Your Body

with **FASCIA THERAPY**

DR. DANIEL FENSTER

HAY HOUSE, INC.
Carlsbad, California • New York City
London • Sydney • New Delhi

Published in the United States by: Hay House, Inc.: www.hayhouse.com®
Published in Australia by: Hay House Australia Pty. Ltd.: www.hayhouse.com.au
Published in the United Kingdom by: Hay House UK, Ltd.: www.hayhouse.co.uk
Published in India by: Hay House Publishers India: www.hayhouse.co.in

Cover design: Howie Severson • *Interior design:* Nick C. Welch • *Indexer:* Joan Shapiro

Interior photos: Page 5: "Structure and Distribution of an Unrecognized Interstitium in Human Tissues," Petros C. Benias et al., Scientific Reports, March 27, 2018, from the Scientfic Reports, May 10, 2018, published by Springer Nature.
Pages 8 and 9: © Fascia Research Society. Photography by Thomas Stephan.
All photos in Part II courtesy of the author.

**Cataloging-in-Publication Data
is on file with the Library of Congress**

Tradepaper ISBN: 978-1-4019-5864-0
E-book ISBN: 978-1-4019-5870-1
Audiobook ISBN: 978-1-4019-5987-6

13   12   11   10   9   8   7   6   5   4
1st edition, June 2020

Printed in the United States of America

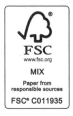

*To my wife, Jan,
and our children,
Zachary, Benjamin,
and Rebekah*

CONTENTS

FOREWORD

When I started working as a health and nutrition coach at Complete Wellness in 2017, I was initially drawn in by their philosophy of being a "one-stop shop" for a wide variety of health concerns. In my years here, I have witnessed truly amazing health outcomes that far exceeded patients' initial expectations. People with chronic pain—many of whom visited doctor after doctor for years, or even decades, with no results—have walked out of our clinic pain-free. Patients who were self-medicating with drugs or alcohol have conquered their addictions as we eased the crippling pain that had devastated their lives. People who could barely walk have returned to biking and jogging. Athletes have not only healed rapidly from injuries but also increased their speed, strength, and agility.

The simple reason behind these success stories is Complete Wellness's patient-focused, holistic approach to health care. As the clinic director, Dr. Fenster guides over a dozen experts to consider each patient as a whole and offer integrative health-care plans rather than singling out and treating symptoms in a piecemeal fashion. In fact, the traditional, symptom-based approach often overlooks a vital aspect of a person's health: your fascia.

If you've never heard of the fascia—or think it's mostly useless bits of connective tissue—get ready to have your eyes opened. Dr. Fenster has shown me that this mysterious organ plays a crucial role in keeping you pain-free, energetic, and happy. That's why I'm thrilled that he's chosen to distill all his knowledge on this important topic in this book, along with the latest research from his interviews with leading experts in the field. Within these pages, you'll find a simple guide to what fascia is, how to assess your own fascial health, and how to support your body with nutrition, at-home therapies, and professional aid.

Stagnant, locked-up fascia can cause a host of problems, including chronic pain, anxiety, sexual problems, and possibly even cancer. Dr. Fenster gives you the knowledge and tools you need to *free your fascia*—either on your own or with the help of experts—to effect healing on a deeper level than you may have ever experienced.

So if you're ready to join the fascia revolution and achieve the peak physical and mental health you deserve . . . read on!

— Liana Werner-Gray,
health researcher, nutrition coach, and best-selling
author of *The Earth Diet* and *Cancer-Free with Food*

PART I

MEET YOUR "MYSTERY" ORGAN

In this section, I'll introduce you to the most important organ you've never heard of—your *fascia*. First, I'll tell you where this organ is (hint: it's everywhere) and why taking care of it is crucial. After that, I'll describe how fascia gets "sick." Finally, I'll offer a quiz you can take to determine how healthy or unhealthy your own fascia is.

CHAPTER 1

WHAT IS FASCIA— AND WHY HAVEN'T YOU HEARD OF IT?

Did you know that there's an organ hiding in plain sight inside your body? In fact, it's the largest organ in your body, running from the top of your head to the soles of your feet. It weaves around and through every single structure in your body. Virtually everything you do, from walking to running a marathon to recovering from an injury, involves this organ.

Yet there's a good chance you've never heard of it.

This organ is your fascia—the least studied, least appreciated organ in the body—and if you've never heard about it, you're not alone. In fact, it's the one organ that doctors barely study in medical school.

It's true that you (and your doctors) do know about bits and pieces of the fascia: for instance, the tendons in your arms, the membranes that surround your brain, and the plantar fascia in your feet. But here's what nearly everyone, including doctors, has missed for centuries: the fascia is *a single, unified organ*—one interconnected, coordinated system!

Why did this big organ remain hidden for centuries? Historically, doctors thought of fascia largely as inert packing material—a biological version of Styrofoam peanuts. Surgeons, for their part, simply cut the fascia out and tossed it away, viewing it as "the stuff that gets in the way of the good stuff." Even anatomists missed the big picture because they generally work on cadavers that are preserved, a process that turns the soft, delicate, water-permeated webwork of the fascia into dry, brittle sticks. When the fascia dies and dries, it takes its secrets with it.

This explains why the fascial system wasn't even recognized in the medical literature until recently. In addition, it explains why your elementary school anatomy lessons taught you about the heart and the liver and the lungs and the brain—but you never heard the word *fascia*.

Now, however, medical science is looking at the fascia with brand-new respect. With the help of computer technology to map fascia's secrets, high-magnification videos taken during surgeries, and autopsies performed on fresh cadavers, we're waking up to the power and importance of the fascia in health and wellness.

Viewing the Living Fascia

In 2015, doctors at Beth Israel Medical Center examined living tissue using a new technology called *probe-based confocal laser endomicroscopy*, which combines a camera-holding probe with a tissue-illuminating laser and sensors that analyze the reflected fluorescent patterns. Using the technology to look at a patient's bile duct, they saw something they didn't expect: a series of interconnected cavities that didn't match any previously known anatomy. Later, when another doctor made slides of the dead tissue, the mysterious cavities had disappeared.

The researchers realized what had happened: the spaces in the biopsy slides, previously dismissed as tears in the tissue, were actually the remains of fluid-filled compartments—fascia—that collapsed after death.[1]

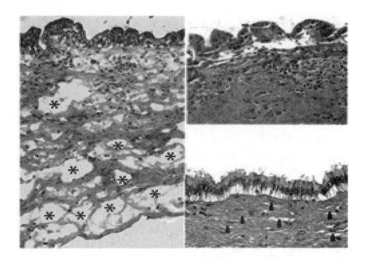

Left: Image of fresh-frozen bile duct; the dark bands are collagen bundles.

Upper right: Image of normally processed and fixed bile duct tissue from the same patient, showing that the spaces have collapsed and the collagen bundles have adhered to each other.

Lower right: Image of the fixed specimen, stained; the thin spaces between collagen layers (arrows) show fluid-filled spaces in the living tissue that are almost completely collapsed.

In recent years, we've discovered that the fascia isn't just inert "filler." Instead, it's a single, interconnected web of tissue that surrounds and penetrates every organ, every muscle, every bone. We now know that fascia runs throughout the entire body and that it's incredibly active biologically.

While fascia is often referred to as *connective tissue*—a phrase that implies that it's simply connecting more important parts of the body—we now understand that it's as critical as any other organ system. This is a new paradigm in medical science, in a field in which new paradigms don't emerge every day, and it's taken even experts in anatomy by surprise.

Sue Hitzmann, creator of the MELT Method (see page 129), told me that she was stunned back in the early 2000s when—after earning a master's degree in exercise science and anatomy at NYU—she participated in a dissection with famed anatomist Gil Hedley and first understood that the fascia was a continuum. "I went back to NYU," she laughs, "and I told them I wanted my money back. I said, 'How can you give me a master's and not even tell me there's another system in the body?'"

As for me, I was in school 35 years ago, long before the fascia revolution began. However, I remember the exact time, early in my training, when my own "aha" moment occurred—well before *fascia* became a mainstream word.

I was in a weekend seminar, learning a soft tissue technique called Nimmo (after Raymond Nimmo, its inventor). Dr. Sheila Laws, the instructor for the seminar, showed us how to hold a trigger point. I had a headache that day, and when someone held a trigger point at the base of my skull, the headache vanished.

Up until that time, I'd focused on the basic tenet of chiropractic: if there is a bone out of alignment, it can irritate a nerve. Adjust the position or mobility of the bone, and you can alleviate the nerve pain. But there's no adjustment involved in Nimmo, which simply involves applying pressure to a trigger point. This opened my eyes to a whole new world, and to the importance of soft tissue—what we now call fascia.

Later, in the mid-'90s, I went to work with Jim and Phil Wharton, who wrote a classic in the bodywork field, *The Whartons' Stretch Book*. As their clinic director, I started to learn about Active Isolated Stretching and the work of Aaron Mattes (see page 70) and incorporated that into my practice. Now I was adding trigger point therapy and stretching to my chiropractic adjustments, and my results just took off.

So I joined the fascia revolution very early on. While I didn't yet understand just how remarkable the fascia is, I knew I was on to something big. Over the next two decades, I began to grasp *how* big when I discovered that as a body-wide organ, the fascia affects how *everything* in the body functions. That's why at Complete Wellness NYC, the top pain-management center in Manhattan, where I am the clinic director, we bring together many different fascia therapies (also known as fascial or myofascial therapies). Specialties include acupuncture, yoga, chiropractic, and more—anything that promotes myofascial healing—because we know that healthy fascia is crucial for a healthy body.

Fortunately, as our knowledge about fascia evolves, more and more health-care practitioners are recognizing this, and they are translating their new knowledge into practice. Professional and Olympic athletes are using fascial treatments both to heal injuries and to take their performance to new levels. Yoga, fascia rolling, and massage therapy are exploding among health-conscious people who want to stay flexible, graceful, and strong. And millions of people who've lived in agony for years because of intractable pain are finding relief via fascial interventions.

Fascia is shaking up the scientific world as well and altering our most fundamental beliefs about the human body. It's revolutionizing our ideas about pain, health, and wellness.

WHAT EXACTLY *IS* FASCIA?

The answer to this question is complex because the fascia has many facets. While it's true that your fascia is one organ, it's an organ with multiple personalities. All fascia contains the same basic components (we'll talk about that in just a minute), but fascial tissue can take on different forms—for instance, sheets, bands, and webs—to perform different jobs.

The shape your fascia chooses for a job basically depends on the amount and direction of the physical pressure and demand you put on it. That's why tendons are tough bands, while the fascia under your skin is weblike and flexible and the fascia around your organs is a little like plastic wrap.

By the way, while you probably didn't realize it, you've already seen lots of fascia when you've looked at animal products. For instance, the silvery-white membranous material on the underside of chicken skin and the thin marbling running through a steak are both fascia. But these are just some of the forms that fascia can take.

The following examples show different forms that fascia can take, depending on the demands placed on them.

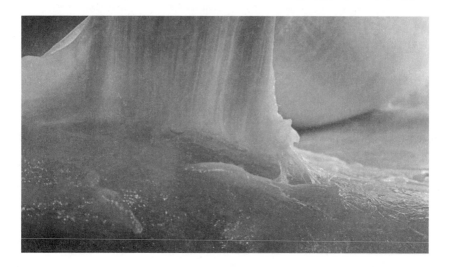

Fascia from a turkey knee
© Fascia Research Society. Photography by Thomas Stephan.

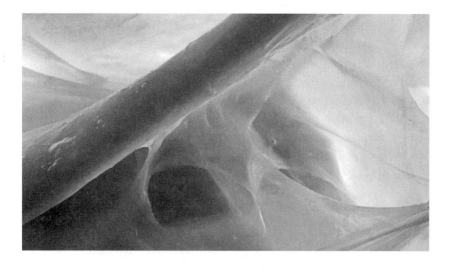

Fascia from a bull leg tendon
© Fascia Research Society. Photography by Thomas Stephan.

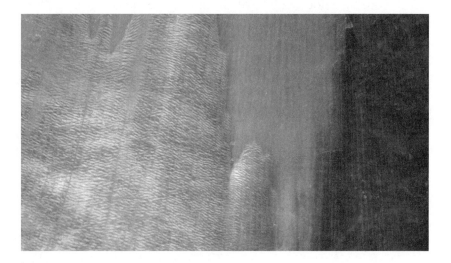

Fascia from a turkey thigh
© Fascia Research Society. Photography by Thomas Stephan.

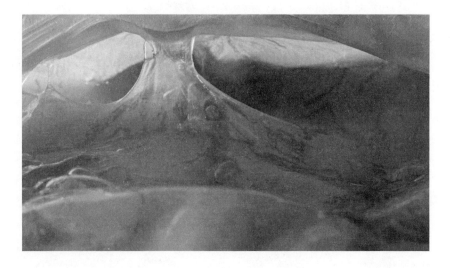

Fascia from a pig brain (meninges)
© Fascia Research Society. Photography by Thomas Stephan.

In your own body, you have multiple layers of fascia. Look under your skin, and you'll find the superficial fascia, a delicate sheath that envelops you from head to toe like a wetsuit.

Go farther in, and you'll find the deep fascia, which surrounds and shapes each muscle and bone and forms the tough, stringy tendons. Finally, you'll reach the visceral fascia—the layers that wrap around your organs, giving them shape and holding them in place.

Now take an even closer look. You'll see that the fascia doesn't just surround your bones and muscles; it *penetrates* them. What's more, it wraps around every cell in your body.

In short, think of your fascia as "bags within bags within bags." Another way to view it is to picture an orange, with its outer peel, its inner sections, and its juice-filled pockets within the sections corresponding to the superficial, deep, and visceral fascia.

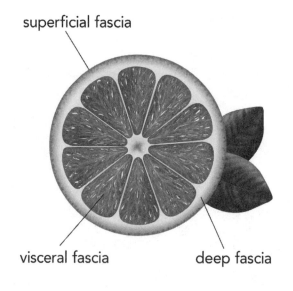

superficial fascia

visceral fascia   deep fascia

Visualization of the layers of fascia

WHAT MAKES UP THE FASCIA?

It's an oversimplification, but you can think of fascia as a liquid-filled mesh made of strings of collagen (the body's most common structural protein) and elastin (a protein that makes tissues snap back after stretching), along with a clear gel called *ground substance.* Picture the fascia as a bath sponge (the collagen and elastin strands) soaked through and through with runny gelatin (the ground substance). The fibers and ground substance make up what's called your *extracellular matrix.*

Within the fascia, you'll also find cells called *fibroblasts.* There aren't many of them compared to the numbers of cells in other tissues, but they're hard workers. Fibroblasts manufacture the collagen, elastin, and other fibers within the fascia, as well as other crucial molecules. As if that job weren't big enough, they're also in charge of cleaning, repairing, and replacing any damaged parts of the fascia—a big task, since about half of the collagen fibers in your fascia get replaced each year. (The building blocks for this replacement process come from your diet, which is why food is so important to fascia health—more about this in Chapters 2 and 7.)

There are other inhabitants of the fascia, but one in particular that I want to mention is hyaluronic acid (yes, the same acid that's in antiwrinkle creams—and the same acid that doctors inject into arthritic knees). Hyaluronic acid, also called hyaluronan, lubricates the ground substance, much like a biological version of WD-40. While it may fight wrinkles on the outside of your skin, it has a much more important job inside your fascia: keeping it from becoming "sticky" so it can glide freely, allowing you to be pain-free and move with strength and grace.

WHAT DOES THE FASCIA DO?

Fascia experts compare the fascia to Superman: at first glance, you think it's just Clark Kent, but when you look more closely, you find out it's a superhero. In fact, far from simply being "packing material," your fascia plays as big a role in your body as your heart, your brain, and your lungs. Here are some of its roles:

It allows the parts of your body to glide over, under, and around each other. Did you ever wonder why you can move with ease and grace—why your skin, bones, muscles, and nerves can all move fluidly when you walk, run, or do any kind of exercise? The reason is that the layers of your fascia glide when you move. In fact, when your fascia is healthy, it can glide up to 75 percent of its length.

It holds everything in place. Fascia anchors and contains your organs, bones, muscles, and blood vessels, making sure they stay where they belong. Without it, your skeleton would just be a pile of bones, and your organs would pool together indiscriminately.

It holds and moves water. Remarkable videos taken by pioneering fascia researcher Dr. Jean-Claude Guimberteau demonstrate that the fascia stores water and transports it throughout the body. In one video, which you can view at www.guimberteau-jc-md.com/en, you can actually see drops of water running down the strands of collagen in the fascia, like dew dripping down a spider web.

It's a body-wide communication network. Your fascia sends every part of your body constant information about your position, your movements, and your internal milieu. Your fascia contains 10 times more sensory nerve endings than your muscles, making it one of the body's most powerful sensory organs. This explains why problems in the fascia are often the real cause of pain blamed solely on your muscles.

It connects every part of your body to every other part of your body. Picture your fascia as a fitted bedsheet. Tug on one corner of the sheet, and every part of the sheet moves. For instance, research by sports medicine specialist Jan Wilke shows that when you move your ankle, the fascia in the back of your upper thigh glides.[2] Stretch your leg, and you affect the fascia of your cervical spine, increasing your ability to move your neck. This is why fascia therapy performed on one part of the body often relieves pain in a distant area, and also why pressure created at one spot on your body can make you feel a sensation in a remote area. The fascia truly embodies the word *holistic*.

We are also discovering that fascia forms "kinetic chains," which are something like movement ropes that run throughout your body. These chains empower multiple parts of your body to move, and to do so with stability, grace, fluidity, energy, and comfort. Our knowledge about the numbers and structure of these chains is still evolving, but dissections of cadavers are revealing where they are and how they function in the body.

This gives us an explanation for many previously mysterious things seen in musculoskeletal care. If something wasn't following a known nerve pattern or a dermatological pattern, we'd say, "Oh, it's in the patient's head." Now that we understand fascia, we have a much deeper understanding of why symptoms happen and how we can address them.

It's a key part of your immune system. Former Harvard researcher Helene Langevin, now at the National Institutes of Health, calls the fascia "the home of the immune system" and believes that understanding it will be a big key to understanding and preventing cancer. In remarkable research, she and her colleagues found that stretching—a technique that optimizes the fascia's function—actually reduces tumor growth in a mouse model of breast cancer (more on this on page 69).[3]

It creates "tensegrity." Why is it that when astronauts go up in space, without gravity and turned upside down, their organs and muscles don't shift around? Why and how does everything stay in place? The answer is *tensegrity*.

Tensegrity creates internal forces that suspend everything in place. In effect, your parts are floating in your fascia, like the fruit my grandmother used to put in gelatin. But tensegrity acts similarly to a magnet, unaffected by gravity.

The bones, organs, and muscles of your body are held in place by your fascia, which acts as your internal support infrastructure. The fascia is able to absorb and disseminate physical stresses throughout its entire structure. For example, when you walk and your foot strikes the ground with each step, your fascia acts as a shock absorber to distribute the impact past just your heel as it strikes the ground. Otherwise, that could hurt!

The term *tensegrity*—a contraction of the words *tension* and *integrity*—was coined by R. Buckminster Fuller, a very popular architect and inventor in the mid- to late 20th century. He saw tensegrity in structures—for instance, his famous "buckyball"—and we are now recognizing that the same tensegrity holds our bodies together and allows us to deal with the physical forces of our everyday lives.

Because of tensegrity, your fascia can store physical energy, just like a spring. Look at the collagen in fascia through a microscope, and you'll see that it has "crimps" in it that allow the fascia to store and release energy as the crimps contract and then stretch. Imagine the forces inside a spring as it recoils and then suddenly explodes when released. This is exactly what happens in your fascia, and it gives you the ability to make ballistic movements such as jumping and throwing.

The tensegrity of your fascia also gives you the ability to remain stable rather than breaking apart when stretching and contorting your body into different positions (think yoga).

It promotes the flow of lymph. Your lymphatic system consists of miles and miles of tubes throughout your body. These tubes carry fluid (lymph) from your tissues to your lymph nodes, which filter toxins, bacteria, cancer cells, and other "garbage" from the lymph and send the cleansed fluid back to your bloodstream. Your muscles and fascia help by pushing lymph through this system as you move—so the healthier your fascia is, the better your lymphatic system performs.

It reacts to stress. Fascia is physically affected by emotional stress, which helps to explain the tightness you feel when you're tense. This is a two-way street because fascial strictures and tightness, in turn, can cause stress and anxiety.

It may influence your emotions and behavior. Exciting new research suggests that fascia doesn't just inform you about where you are but also helps to tell you *how* you are.[4] It appears to play a role in providing the brain with *interoceptive* information, or information about your physiological state. This information—for instance, how hot or cold you are, how hungry or thirsty you are, how well (or unwell) you feel, even your level of sexual arousal—has an emotional as well as a sensory component. Abnormal interoception has been linked to a wide range of conditions including irritable bowel syndrome, eating disorders, anxiety, and depression (more on this in my interview with Dr. Robert Schleip on page 23).

In short, fascia doesn't play a small role in your body. It plays a *huge* role, and that's why it deserves the respect it's now starting to receive. Thousands of doctors and therapists around the world are now targeting the fascia in order to relieve people's pain, enhance their performance, and improve their lives.

Note: As you've seen, the fascia connects and interacts with every part of your body, never acting in isolation. As a result, when we treat the fascia, we're also affecting other structures—in particular the muscles. (Remember that fascia both surrounds and runs through the muscles.) That is why the term *myofascial* (the root *myo* means "muscle") is used interchangeably in this book with the term *fascial*.

Tom Myers: Fascia as Fabric

Tom Myers, author of *Anatomy Trains* and co-author of *Fascial Release for Structural Balance*, has revolutionized the fascia world with a series of dissections showing how fascia forms "trains" within the body. Recently, I asked him about the evolving awareness of fascia as a system.

How do you view fascia?

Fascia is the fabric that weaves our 70 trillion cells together. You may think that you are you, but you are not—you are a community of 70 trillion cells. They are wet, they're greasy, and something has to hold them together. So they are woven together in the fascia, which is a sinewy fabric that goes between all of the cells.

Why is this concept of fascia so new?

The reason is that fascia is the context for all other body activity. We didn't see it because it was an environment. We didn't see it because we are goldfish, and we don't understand about the water in the bowl. We live in the water, but we don't understand it.

I did a lot of dissections in earlier years, and we just tried to get the connecting tissue out of the way so we could see the "interesting" stuff. Well, we now understand that we need to pay attention to the properties and the physiology of the fascia itself.

How much awareness of fascia is there in the medical community?

The idea of fascia is rapidly becoming more and more acknowledged. However, I must say, if I talk to general practitioners, they don't understand what I'm talking about. Their last encounter with fascia was in a gross anatomy class dissecting a formaldehyded body, in which the fascia had been fixed [which turns it dry and brittle]. So if I say to them, "I'm changing the fascia," they say, "You can't change the fascia."

But if I talk to orthopedists who are working with living fascia every day, they understand what I'm doing right away.

What kinds of changes do you see in patients after a bodywork session?

We take photographs before and after sessions, and we can see that the knees of a bowlegged person are closer together or that the curvatures in a person's back have indeed balanced out with each other. It's great when we can make those biomechanical changes, which make life easier for people.

THE PHYSICAL BENEFITS OF FASCIA THERAPY

As you can guess, procedures involving the fascia—the largest organ in the body, and one that influences every other structure— can have far-reaching effects. The more we learn about the fascia, the more we're discovering just how amazing these effects can be.

One of the most life-changing results of fascia therapy, of course, is pain relief. In our own clinic, we've helped thousands of patients get quick relief from pain, often after years or even decades of suffering. What's more, we're not the only people getting these results; in fact, the medical literature is filled with case studies of therapy relieving pain stemming from diabetic neuropathy, back problems, knee surgery, hip injuries, temporomandibular joint disorder, migraines, or carpal tunnel syndrome, to name just a sampling.[5] More and more doctors are discovering that simple, noninvasive fascial therapies can free pain sufferers from the need for dangerous opioid painkillers or invasive surgeries.

Athletes, too, are using fascial treatments to recover from injuries—and beyond that, they're using them to dramatically "up their games." Michael Phelps, who won six Olympic medals in 2016, caused a stir when he arrived at the pool covered in circular marks caused by "cupping"—a form of fascia therapy that I'll talk about later. Other fans of fascial approaches range from Stanley Cup winner Valtteri Filppula of the Detroit Red Wings to Buffalo Bills linebacker Lorenzo Alexander to Olympic figure skater Patrick Chan.

However, it's not just pain sufferers or athletes who are turning to fascial therapies. Thousands of papers in the medical literature show that treating the fascia can have wide-ranging benefits, including the following:

- **Lower blood pressure.** Multiple studies show that massage, which releases the fascia, can cause significant decreases in blood pressure.[6] In addition, new research shows that Kinesio taping—a simple form of fascia therapy I'll discuss in Chapter 8—can lower blood pressure and reduce cardiac vagal tone in people with hypertension, with benefits lasting at least five days after each session.[7]

- **Better sleep.** Research shows that fascial release via massage can improve the quality of sleep for both children and adults and can improve sleep in infants by easing symptoms of colic.[8]

- **Fewer premenstrual symptoms.** Massage therapy can enhance mood and decrease premenstrual pain. In one study, for instance, researchers assigned 24 people with premenstrual dysphoric disorder to a massage therapy group or a relaxation therapy group.[9] They found that the massage group showed decreases in anxiety, depressed mood, and pain immediately after the first and last massage sessions. Other effects of massage therapy included reductions in water retention and overall menstrual distress.

- **An easier pregnancy.** Research shows that mothers receiving massage therapy have shorter labors, a shorter hospital stay, less predelivery anxiety, and less postpartum depression.[10] Remarkably, one study showed that women who received massage therapy had labors that were on average *three hours* shorter, with less need for medication.[11]

- **Better bladder control.** Doctors report that fascial release is an effective treatment for interstitial cystitis and urinary urgency.[12]

- **Relief from gastroesophageal reflux disease (GERD).** Researchers in Spain performed either myofascial release therapy or a sham therapy on 30 patients with GERD. They report that myofascial release therapy led to fewer GERD symptoms, a better quality of life, and reduced use of proton pump inhibitors such as Nexium, Losec, and Prevacid.[13]

- **Relief from dizziness.** Dry needling, a form of fascia therapy, can help to relieve cervical vertigo—one of the most common forms of chronic dizziness.[14]

- **Weight loss.** When you're flexible and pain-free, exercise is easy rather than difficult, so you move more and burn more fat. Healing your fascia also improves your circulation and makes it easier for your body to flush out toxins, boosting your metabolism and promoting weight loss.

- **Better posture.** Fascia therapy releases the triggers that distort your posture, fixing imbalances caused by anything from "wallet butt" (from sitting on a fat wallet) to "toddler back" (from carrying kids on one hip). It can even help with more serious posture problems; for instance, studies show that people with scoliosis (a sideways curve of the spine) or postural hyperkyphosis (an exaggerated front-to-back curve of the upper spine) have less spinal curvature after fascia therapy.[15]

Aaron Mattes, a mentor of mine and the inventor of a powerful fascia therapy called Active Isolated Stretching (AIS—see page 70), recently shared two examples of the amazing effects of his therapy on severe scoliosis.

One case involved a young woman who'd graduated from college but was unable to fulfill her dream of going to veterinary school because of her severe scoliosis. "We worked for one week—five days," Mattes told me. "At the end of the five days, she was straight as a string. Her scoliosis was completely gone." The second case involved an elderly woman with scoliosis so severe that her back and head were bent approximately 45 to 60 degrees to the right. Mattes said that after therapy, her back was completely straight.

While most cases of scoliosis will not respond this dramatically (and some may not respond at all), thousands of people may be able to forego painful surgeries or uncomfortable back braces and reduce their scoliosis with simple, noninvasive interventions like Mattes's.

Case Study 1: The Weekend Warrior

One of our patients—we'll call him DJ—was diagnosed with severe carpal tunnel syndrome by his general practitioner and referred to an orthopedic surgeon. DJ knew he needed help for his crippling problem, but the thought of surgery scared him, so he came to our clinic seeking a better solution.

DJ liked to work out on the weekends, and his favorite form of exercise was cycling. He spent so much time leaning on his wrists on his bike that he developed pain in his right wrist and fingers, extending into his elbow, shoulder, neck, and even sometimes the back of his head. Spending long hours in front of his computer at work only made matters worse.

DJ's symptoms did indeed resemble carpal tunnel syndrome, but they were much more extensive. When questioned, DJ also revealed that he had tightness in his face and jaw.

Looking at his pain patterns from a classic neurological viewpoint, it was hard to make a clear diagnosis. However, through the fascial lens, it made perfect sense.

The deep and superficial front and back arm lines are fascial kinetic chains that run from the fingers up to the head. DJ had contractures and adhesions in these lines, restricting proper function of the muscles, entrapping the nerves, and sending pain along that entire line. Based on the resulting pain pattern, it was easy to determine the correct treatment for him.

DJ began a soft tissue–based care plan involving two visits per week for four weeks and cut back on his biking during that time. At the end of the plan, he was completely pain-free and happily cycling again.

Case Study 2: The Reeling Runner

MM was a long-distance runner for many years. In addition, he sat for long hours in front of a computer at work. As a result, he developed a round-shouldered slump, and his head lurched forward. This posture puts destructive forces on the fascia and other soft tissues of the whole body, especially from the waist up.

MM decided that he wanted a stronger core, so he began a course of sit-ups. Unfortunately, MM's poor form as he lifted his head upward and contracted his abs only made the stress on his body worse.

Around this time, MM began to have dizzy spells. When I examined him, it was clear that his problem involved the fascia. In the fascial network, there are mechanoreceptors (which respond to pressure, stretching, gravity, and other mechanical stimuli) and proprioceptors (which tell us where we are in space), and these help us to determine our posture in our three-dimensional world. When these receptors receive overwhelmingly disruptive information, the system can go haywire and create symptoms such as dizziness.

To solve MM's problem, we had to treat his fascial aberrations, reorient his nervous system, correct his posture, stretch his chest muscles, and strengthen the muscles and fascia in his upper back and neck. Interestingly, this new information was disruptive to his old norm. He went through another short period of dizziness as his body reoriented to his new, better function.

After a relatively short course of care, MM was back to running, in great form and with improved posture. Shoulders back and head high, he felt great.

THE MENTAL BENEFITS OF FASCIA THERAPY

In addition to affecting your body, fascial treatments can have a dramatic effect on your state of mind. Tight, tense fascia causes you to breathe shallowly, contributing to anxiety and even panic attacks.[16] Therapy releases the fascia, allowing you to breathe deeply and easily and calming anxiety.

Another possible reason for the mood-enhancing effects of fascia therapy is that your fascia contains receptors for *endocannabinoids*—substances produced by your body that have biological effects similar to the effects of marijuana.[17] One study showed that after subjects received osteopathic manipulation, the serum level of anandamide—a neurotransmitter classified as an endocannabinoid—increased by 168 percent.[18]

Therapies that affect the fascia can also ease depression. In one study of 755 people with moderate or severe depression, researchers found that acupuncture lowered scores on a 27-point scale of depressive symptoms from an average of 16 to 9 over the course of the study.[19] One in three patients was no longer depressed after three months of acupuncture, compared to one in five among the control group.

□ □ □

In short, taking good care of your fascia can make you feel stronger, healthier, and happier from head to toe—which makes perfect sense, since the fascia is a head-to-toe organ. So pampering your fascia is a very smart move, and in these pages, I'll tell you exactly how to do it.

Before we talk about how to optimize the health of your fascia, however, let's talk about something else: how things can go wrong for your fascia in the first place.

Dr. Robert Schleip: "Gut Feelings" and More

Dr. Robert Schleip is the director of the Fascia Research Group and one of the world's foremost fascia researchers. Currently, he and his colleagues are exploring a new and exciting facet of fascia: its effects on interoception.

What is interoception?

Interoception basically means body sensations linked to physiological and emotional needs, not so much to biomechanical requirements. It's less related to how we move—*How fast am I walking? Where is my shoulder in space?*—and it's also less related to posture and movement. That is proprioception.

Examples of interoception include hunger or warmth or tingling. These are body sensations for sure, and all of them originate not from myelinated nerve endings but from free nerve endings—for example, the free nerve endings you have in your gut. So a gut feeling that something happening around you feels wrong is usually interoception.

How can fascial work impact interoception?

If you do visceral fascial work, you can feel its impact on interoception immediately.

When you do gentle osteopathic or Rolfing work in the visceral connective tissues and you cause an increase in peristalsis [the constriction and relaxation of the intestines that moves food through the body] that you feel immediately under your hands, then you have influenced the autonomic nervous system—and this happens via the stretch receptors in the visceral connective tissue. So any myofascial work focusing on visceral connective tissue most likely is impacting more on interoception than on proprioception.

Certain pathologies go along with a disturbed interoception, not so much with a disturbed proprioception. If someone has chronic low back pain, it is mostly proprioception that is dysfunctional, not interoception. So if people have chronic low back pain, doing Rolfing movement or Iyengar yoga or Feldenkrais, where you specifically ask people to pay attention to proprioception, is very, very powerful. However, if you have someone with eating disorders or somebody with post-traumatic stress disorder, in those cases focusing on proprioception may be the wrong primary goal. It may be useful somehow, but it's probably not making a major difference.

How can a therapist focus on interoception?

You may ask the client, "Do you feel any kind of sensational difference? Is the leg heavier, or is it lighter?" Of course, that doesn't mean the leg weighs more or less when you weigh it on a scale. But it feels heavier, or it feels lighter, or it feels more spacious, and these are sensations that are linked to interoception.

What is the emotional component of interoception?

Interoception always has an affective coloring. If you change proprioception, and you ask me, "Is 90 degrees on the elbow more pleasant than 60 degrees?" I often cannot tell you. I feel a difference, but they are both okay. However, if you change the temperature in the bathtub, you can always say whether it's getting more pleasant or less pleasant. Interoception always involves more well-being or less well-being.

I think if you're getting bodywork, it should be not only to improve how well you can control your body so you're perfectly symmetrical and look straight in the mirror but should also focus on embodiment and feeling at home in your body.

How have you seen bodywork therapies evolve as we've learned more about the fascia?

In Feldenkrais [a form of bodywork], we used to focus on the skeleton. We said, "Forget your muscles, forget your connective tissue." Connective tissue in Moshe Feldenkrais's time was treated in general with as little relative respect as you would treat the wrapping of a Christmas present; we'd focus on the present and not on the wrapping. We'd focus attention on the bones—"Do you feel the movement of your humerus in relationship to the shoulder blade?"

However, when you focus solely on the bones, your body consists of 200 parts. If you focus on fascia, you still can go into the shoulder joint, but the shoulder joint is not a fragmented part. It becomes just one aspect of a body-wide interconnected tensional network.

For me, this is a great contribution of modern bodyworkers who come from a somatic perspective, and it is where fascia makes a very big contribution. When you focus on interoception as well as on fascial proprioception, you feel that your body is not just many different pieces put together by a great engineer but is one organic unity—one living person. A person who has been stimulated on that level of somatic perception may more likely feel the connectedness in their body and their sense of aliveness—as a bubbling life energy—and they're glad in the morning that they woke up in this living body.

CHAPTER 2

WHY GOOD
FASCIA GOES BAD

Free fascia is a beautiful thing. It glides with ease, so you can move and do so painlessly, gracefully, and joyfully. It's springy and resilient, so it energizes and supports you. It makes you happier and healthier all over, and research hints that it's even a powerful tool in your cancer-fighting arsenal.

That's why keeping your fascia healthy—or getting it back in shape, if it's congested, stagnant, or locked up right now—needs to be a top priority in your health regimen. Luckily, there are steps you can take to set your fascia free and keep it that way. No matter how old you are or how long your fascia has been dysfunctional, you can make things better—and there's a chance that you can recover completely from chronic pain or disability and achieve wellness and optimal performance.

However, before I talk about healing your fascia, I want to talk about what's hurting it. Here are the top eight villains in this story:

VILLAIN 1: TOO LITTLE MOVEMENT

Think for a minute about how our earliest ancestors lived. They spent hours and hours every day bending, stretching, walking, lifting, and throwing. They ran away from predators and chased after prey. They danced, fought, and hunted for food. In a thousand different ways, they moved their bodies from sunup to sundown.

Things are very different for us today. No matter what we do for a living, most of us spend hours each day sitting in front of a computer, sitting in a car, and making the same limited, repetitive motions day after day. After that, we spend more hours on the couch in the evening, binge-watching Netflix or texting friends.

Unfortunately, the cliché "use it or lose it" is never truer than when it comes to fascia. That's because when fascia doesn't move, it dries out, stiffens, gets sticky, and even becomes toxic. In fact, lack of movement is number one on our list of fascia villains because it's such a common issue and because, short of injury or overuse, it's the worst thing that can happen to your fascia.

To understand why your fascia craves constant movement, recall my sponge analogy. Think of your fascia as a sponge filled with water that gets a little dirty over time, and imagine squeezing that sponge so the water runs out. Then picture dipping the sponge in a bucket so it soaks up clean, fresh water.

Things work much the same way in your fascia. Over time, the fascia accumulates toxins such as lactic acid and pyruvic acid. These are normal by-products of muscle function—a little like the exhaust from a car—that damage the fascia if they don't get cleaned out. "Squeezing the sponge" by moving your body allows the fascia to replace old water with new.

Another good analogy is a pump. When you move, the resulting pressure on your fascia pumps water out of it, sweeping out toxins along with it. Then, when you rest your fascia, fresh water gets pumped back into it, cleansing and hydrating it and feeding it the nutrients it needs. This move-and-rest cycle is the key to keeping your fascia refreshed, well-fed, and fluid enough to glide easily.

When your fascia doesn't move regularly—for instance, when you sit in front of a computer all day, every day—very bad things happen to it. As Dr. Brent Anderson, an expert on Pilates, describes it, "When we put ourselves in a position, our fascia is just printing the position we're in. So if we're always sitting, then our fascia looks like sitting fascia."

In an eye-opening study back in 2002, researchers immobilized the body parts of rats for three weeks.[1] The result was shocking: the elegant webbing of the fascia became tangled, matted, and thickened, with an excess of collagen threads going in every direction. And that's just in a few weeks, so imagine what years of inactivity can do.

There are two lessons here. The first lesson is that "motion is lotion," and the fascia needs to move in many different directions every day. The second lesson is that resting after you move is key. That's when you allow the water to rush back into your thirsty fascial sponge.

When you exercise, keep these important tips in mind:

- **Use your full range of motion.** Picture a train constantly running back and forth on the same four feet of track. That part of the track will stay smooth and shiny, but the rest will get rusty from disuse. Similarly, if you only make small movements most of the time, going beyond those limits will be painful. Instead, stretch and exercise to your limits on a regular basis.

- **Mix it up.** We tend to label ourselves as runners or swimmers or basketball players and to stick to one sport. However, the more ways in which you move your body, the healthier your fascia will be. That's one reason why, after decades as a runner, I tackled a triathlon. By adding biking and swimming, I took my workout routine to a whole new level.

  In addition, I mix things up as much as possible even when I'm doing one activity, like weightlifting. I might do high repetitions with a low weight or fewer repetitions with a heavier weight.

- **Work both sides.** If you're a golfer or a baseball player, for instance, occasionally swing your club or bat from the opposite side. This will help to prevent fascial constrictions.

VILLAIN 2: INJURIES

Fascia is everywhere in your body, so any time you injure your-self—whether you roll an ankle or wrench your back while lifting a heavy box—you damage your fascia. Surgeries leave their mark on your fascia as well, and pregnancy and delivery can lead to fascial trauma, sometimes causing chronic pain or incontinence.[2]

Not every injury is a crisis for your fascia. Because it's normally very resilient, small injuries aren't such a big deal (unless you continue to reinjure an area by overusing it—something I'll talk about shortly). But a large injury, or even a smaller one if your fascia is unhealthy, can lead to long-term trouble. That's because the collagen fibers in the injured area may begin to grow in a tangled, crisscrossing pattern as they attempt to patch the damaged spot. As a result, knots and adhesions can form, trapping toxins, restricting your movement, and leading to loss of function and even extreme pain.

Also, as I mentioned in Chapter 1, the fascia is like a fitted bed-sheet: tug on one part, and you affect every other part. That is why, when you injure one area of your fascia, pain, tingling, or weakness can appear in a distant area. (Remember the kinetic chains I talked about earlier, which link distant parts of the fascia.)

What's more, you'll begin to compensate for a fascial injury by holding or moving *other* parts of your body in a different way. The longer an injury lasts, the more you will compensate for it and the more symptoms you will experience throughout your body.

For instance, I experienced a traumatic eye injury when I was four years old that has impacted me throughout my life. When I was on a hike with my family, a thorn went into my left eye after a branch snapped into my face. Even after multiple surgeries and treatment, my vision on that side is so fuzzy that I use a slight rotation and a head tilt to bring my good eye more center. In compensating for my vision, I've established a habit that significantly affects the fascia and muscles in my neck.

VILLAIN 3: OVERUSE

I've talked about how critical it is to move if you want to keep your fascia hydrated and healthy. However, one type of movement—*overuse*—can seriously damage the fascia. That's why performing the same movement over and over again during the day, and doing it day after day—whether it's kicking a football, scanning groceries, or lifting heavy boxes at work—can lead to problems.

When most of us think of trauma, we think of a sprained ankle or a torn meniscus or a broken bone. This is *gross* trauma, usually caused by a fall or an accident. However, chronic bad posture and repeated actions can cause very minute tears in your fascia, called *microtraumas*. While these aren't as severe as a major trauma, they definitely can have long-term effects—especially if the same microtrauma is repeated many times over a long period.

As a result of our careers, my wife and I have both experienced problems due to overuse. As a chiropractor, I spend hours each weekday bending over a table. As a result, I chronically restrict some areas of my fascia and need to be vigilant about freeing these areas. My wife, Jan, for her part, used to sling a heavy bag of yoga supplies over her left shoulder while she walked from client to client in the city. As a result, she developed pain in her neck, shoulder, and upper back. These days, she's learned to carry a smaller bag and switch her bag from arm to arm.

Overuse can involve any part of your body. If you deliver packages all day, you can create microtraumas in the fascia in your arms, legs, or back. If you carry a baby on your hip for hours each day, you can stress the fascia in your hip, side, back, arms, and neck. But there's one specific form of overuse—the "text neck" that's a hallmark of smartphone users—that's especially problematic these days, particularly among young people.

When you sit or stand in a hunched posture with your head forward, as you do when you're texting, you place a huge strain on your myofascial system. Spinal surgeon Kenneth Hansraj notes, "An adult head weighs 10 to 12 pounds in the neutral position. As the head tilts forward the forces seen by the neck surge to 27 pounds at

15 degrees, 40 pounds at 30 degrees, 49 pounds at 45 degrees and 60 pounds at 60 degrees."[3] In other words, your neck is supporting the equivalent of a 40- to 60-pound bowling ball whenever you bend your head to send a text message.

The fascia and muscles in your neck and back can handle this load for a little while and still recover. However, these days, Dr. Hansraj says, "people spend an average of two to four hours a day with their heads tilted over reading and texting on their smartphones and devices. Cumulatively this is 700 to 1,400 hours a year of excess stresses seen about the cervical spine."[4] That's serious overuse—and it's why dozens of patients arrive at our clinic each week with headaches, back pain, and neck pain due to texting.

VILLAIN 4: DEHYDRATION

Exercise is the best way to pump liquid into your fascia. However, your body can't rehydrate the fascia if there isn't enough moisture in your body to begin with. Unfortunately, many of us are cheating our fascia of water, with research suggesting that up to 75 percent of us are chronically dehydrated.[5]

One big problem, of course, is that we don't drink enough water. But that's only part of the picture. We also work in artificially heated and cooled buildings that dry us out. We take long flights in airplanes with virtually no humidity. We eat too much processed food, which requires more water to process, and too few water-rich fruits and vegetables. We take medications, from Sudafed to Tylenol to Xanax, that steal water from our bodies. And our epidemic of obesity is taking a toll, since people who are obese are at higher risk for dehydration.[6]

Even using our phones, computers, or tablets can affect us in surprising ways. In their fascinating book, *Quench: Beat Fatigue, Drop Weight, and Heal Your Body through the New Science of Optimum Hydration*, Dana Cohen, M.D. (a colleague of mine at Complete Wellness NYC), and Gina Bria say, "Heat dehydrates. Think of all those lights and electronic devices that warm up by just being on. Have you ever noticed how hot your computer can get, or even your phone?"

In addition, they say, "All that sitting and slumping over keyboards and phones suppresses and restricts the vital flow of fluid throughout our whole system."

Also, while it's still speculative, there's mounting evidence that our devices dehydrate us in another way: via the electromagnetic frequencies that blanket our bodies every day. According to one prestigious research group, "Bioeffects can occur *in the first few minutes* at levels associated with cell and cordless phone use. Bioeffects can also occur from just minutes of exposure to mobile phone masts (cell towers), WI-FI, and wireless utility 'smart' meters that produce whole-body exposure."[7] The researchers note that this electro-smog interferes with normal body processes and disrupts our metabolism—and anything that affects the body in these ways almost certainly affects our hydration, because it takes extra hydration to repair damage to the body.

In short, modern life is a perfect storm of insults that dry out our fascia. As a result, we need more water than ever before—but the vast majority of us aren't getting it.

Dana Cohen, M.D.: How to Keep Your Fascia Hydrated in a Dry World

Dana Cohen, M.D., is an internist who specializes in helping people heal using lifestyle interventions, diet, and other non-drug approaches. She is a member of our staff at Complete Wellness and is the co-author (with Gina Bria) of *Quench: Beat Fatigue, Drop Weight, and Heal Your Body through the New Science of Optimum Hydration*.

What's the link between hydration and fascia?

A few years ago, a plastic surgeon named Jean-Claude Guimberteau [see page 12] decided to put an electron microscope camera under the skin of a living person. What he saw is that fascia is actually a delivery system of fluid.

We'd only looked at fascia from dried, desiccated cadavers before that, and we'd thought that hydration gets moved solely via blood and lymph. So this is a whole new delivery system of hydration that we've never really known about. The idea that you have to move your joints to lubricate them is intuitive, but now we have real reasons why. It's the fascia that's moving. And with massage, you're not just breaking up fascia, you're moving fluid.

This is yet another reason why sitting is the new smoking. When you're sitting, you're squelching that delivery system of fluid to your extremities.

Hydration runs every single system in our bodies, including detoxification. If we're not hydrated enough, we're not functioning at optimal performance. That's why it's my opinion—and the opinion of many others—that hydration is the first and most important step we need to take in preventing and treating chronic illness. Before you start a new diet or plan, you have to know how to hydrate first.

How can people know if they have dehydration?

Let me first say that I'm not talking about overt dehydration, where you need to be hospitalized because you need an IV. I'm talking about a subclinical, low-grade dehydration that almost all of us experience at some point. There's no lab test you can do, so we have to look at you clinically. The biggest thing you can do is to look at the color of your urine. You want it to be a straw color, not too clear and not too dark. (One note here: if you are taking B vitamins, they can turn your urine neon yellow.) Also, you should be getting up to urinate every two to three hours during the day.

To me, the most common symptoms of low-grade dehydration are afternoon fatigue and brain fog. Most people will go to grab sugar, thinking, "Oh, my blood sugar's dropping." More often than not, it's low hydration.

We know that the fascia is the vehicle that moves the hydration. But what happens to the fascia when hydration is low?

Our fascia is where we hold most of our water. When we're in a low-grade, subclinical dehydrated state, the body will take water from wherever it can be taken—including the fascia—in order to feed our brain first.

When these dips in hydration happen in our fascia, toxins accumulate, inflammation accumulates, and our joints are more prone to pain, stiffness, and injury because of the inflammation and the toxins that aren't getting flushed out like they should be.

What is the "gel water" in our cells that you talk about in your book?

We've only known water to exist as liquid, ice, and vapor. Now we know, based on the work of Dr. Gerald Pollack and his water research lab in Seattle, that there's a "fourth phase," gel water. He calls this phase H_3O_2. Gel water is in the state that's believed to exist in our cells. It's also that state that's found in nature in plants.

Think about how desert plants like aloe hydrate. When you open a leaf of aloe, gel falls out of it. That's water in gel form. Similarly, when you add liquid to chia seeds, they form a little gel around them that makes it possible to make a chia pudding with them. Also, think about cucumber seeds, which have that little gel around them.

This is why the best way to stay hydrated is to drink a green smoothie every day. If you've never tried this, you will absolutely notice a difference within a few days—in your energy, your fluidity, and your ease of movement. [See page 136 for Dr. Cohen's smoothie suggestions.]

Can you think of a case study that exemplified to you the power of hydration?

Let me tell you about Betty. She was really interesting.

When Betty came to see me, she was walking like an old woman. She was in her early fifties, and in so much pain all over from fibromyalgia. She was miserable, and she was drinking a lot of wine to numb the pain at night and put her to sleep.

I did my workup on Betty, sent her home, and told her to start the Quench plan. She couldn't even walk for exercise, so I had her do some simple shoulder lifts and head bobbing. She started drinking a green smoothie every day, having a big glass of water in the morning with electrolytes and eating a little bit differently to increase her hydration.

She came back three weeks later, literally jumping up and down at the front desk, screaming, "I feel so much better!" And over the course of the next one to two years, she completely turned things around. She is sober, and she's like a different person. She's really changed her life.

Good hydration was that little push that got the ball rolling. That's why I say that hydration needs to be the first step in any plan.

VILLAIN 5: STRESS

Stress makes your fascia tight, and tight fascia, in turn, increases your stress. It's a vicious circle in which millions of people in today's high-pressure world are trapped.

Living in New York City, I can see this problem is nearly universal among the patients and clients of my clinic. When we're working with them, we can clearly see the effects of stress on their fascia. It shows in their faces, their necks, and their jaws. We can see it in their posture and feel it in the form of fascial tightness, knots, and restrictions.

We can release this tension via fascia therapy or yoga, but that's just one part of the process. In addition, they—and you, if you're under stress—need to actively take control of stress using techniques like the ones I'll outline in Chapter 7.

VILLAIN 6: AGING

We can't do much about getting older—and, as the saying goes, it beats the alternative. However, it's important to realize that aging plays a big role in the health of your fascia and that as you get older, you need to get even more serious about your fascial fitness.

There's no getting around the fact that fascia changes as we age. It gets stiff, it breaks down, and it dries out. (Fascia expert Thomas Myers likes to raise the question, "Are you aging or just drying out?")

However, there are ways you can fight back. One enemy of fascia is gravity, which pulls us down and compresses the fascia; the older we get, the more gravity wins this battle. To slow this process, you can do activities, including stretching, yoga, and tai chi, that counter the pull of gravity and also pump more water into the fascia. Eating right and reducing your exposure to toxins can slow the fascial aging process, too—which brings us to our next two villains.

VILLAIN 7: A BAD DIET

What you eat can have a huge effect on your fascia, for good or bad—and today, many people are loading up on fascia-damaging foods and, at the same time, starving their fascia of the nutrients it needs.

Let's talk about the bad foods first. The biggest culprit here is sugar, which combines with protein in your body to form molecules called *advanced glycation end products*, or AGEs. AGEs are very bad news because these destructive molecules cause the collagen fibers in your fascia (and elsewhere in your body) to "cross-link," making them stiff and misshapen and making it impossible for the body to repair them. The damage caused by AGEs reduces your fascia's ability to glide and slide; one study of the effects of AGEs on tendons found that "the main mechanical effect of AGEs is a loss of tissue viscoelasticity driven by matrix-level loss of fiber-fiber sliding."[8] (Translation: the tendons get "sticky.")

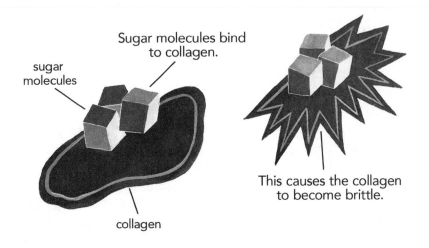

The process of glycation

But it's not just too much sugary food that damages the fascia; it's also too little good food. One of the biggest mistakes you can make when it comes to your fascia is to eat too few natural, unprocessed foods that help build, protect, and replace collagen. We'll talk more about these foods in Chapter 7, but one group of foods that deserves special mention here is foods high in vitamin C.

Vitamin C is required to form procollagen, which your body uses to make different types of collagen. Vitamin C is actually a "rate-limiting" factor for collagen, which means that when the vitamin C runs out, your collagen production line shuts down. And remember: fascia is largely collagen fibers soaked with water. So if you're shorting yourself on vitamin C, your fascia will take a big hit.

Scurvy: A Collagen Deficiency Disease

Here's a little historical trivia that ties in with the topic of fascia and diet. Scurvy—the debilitating and even deadly disease that once struck down thousands of sailors—is a disease caused by the body's inability to replace broken-down collagen with newly made collagen due to a lack of vitamin C. Eventually, sailors started getting a daily ration of citrus juice, which solved the problem.

You don't see people dying of scurvy these days because we get at least marginal amounts of vitamin C in our diets—but millions of us aren't getting enough to optimize our collagen production, and our fascia is suffering as a result.

VILLAIN 8: TOXINS

Like every other organ in your body, your fascia suffers when you're exposed to toxins in food, air, or water. Toxins inflame your body, damage your cells, dehydrate you, and deplete you of nutrients, and all of this impacts the fascia.

Nutritionist Liana Werner-Gray says, "Toxins break down collagen. Imagine the fascia is like a string of pasta, flexible and durable. Then pour some poison (toxins) on it, and the pasta becomes weak and dissolves and becomes separated, no longer holding itself together."

Luckily, even in a dirty world, there are ways you can keep this exposure to a minimum. In Chapter 7, I'll tell you about some easy steps that can slash your body burden of toxic chemicals.

There's one form of toxic exposure that I want to single out here, and that's smoking. Smoking is particularly brutal on the fascia because it lowers the supply of oxygen and the amounts of nutrients it gets. This is one reason why people who smoke are nearly three times more likely than nonsmokers to have chronic back pain, and why they have more trouble healing after surgery.[9]

□ □ □

As you can see, a variety of different insults—from fast-food lunches to injuries to a sedentary lifestyle to excessive texting—can take a toll on your fascia. Over time, these insults can add up, leaving you stiff, inflexible, or even in chronic pain.

The good news is that you can free that tight, knotted, "sticky" fascia—and you can do it in simple, safe, and noninvasive ways. Often, you can do it on your own; other times, you can do it with the help of a professional. In the next chapter, I'll help you decide if the do-it-yourself or professional approach is right for you.

Dr. Antonio Stecco:
When Fascia Is a Family Affair

Physiatrist Antonio Stecco, M.D., is a member of the fascia community's most prominent family. His father, physical therapist Luigi Stecco, was one of the first professionals to recognize the importance of the fascia and is the originator of a powerful technique called Fascial Manipulation®. His sister, orthopedic surgeon Carla Stecco, M.D., is the author of the groundbreaking book *Functional Atlas of the Human Fascial System*. He himself has written many works, including the paradigm-changing book *Fascial Manipulation for Musculoskeletal Pain* (co-authored with his sister).

Among them, the Steccos and their team of researchers have published more than 150 scientific papers. Antonio's own work focuses primarily on understanding the anatomy of fascia, and particularly the relationship between fascia and muscle.

Dr. Stecco's interest in the fascia began early. "I was a sports guy," he says, "and I had major and minor injuries. My father was treating me, and I saw the results. So I was curious: What is the mechanism that leads to these results?" That curiosity led him, in time, to join his father and become one of the world's most prominent fascia researchers. He has worked for more than 10 years in the Department of Human Anatomy and Physiology at the University of Padua, doing more than 100 cadaver dissections to uncover the secrets of the fascia.

"We started with anatomy," Dr. Stecco says. "You know, what is fascia? Then we moved on into the biomechanics—how fascia can transmit loads, how fascia can glide on the muscle. And then we moved into histology—how the cells produce the lubricant, the hyaluronan, to permit the gliding between the different layers of fascia and between fascia and muscle. Now we're doing research that's even more clinical, in order to understand how this hyaluronan can change. It can cause an increase in intracellular matrix viscosity, reducing lubrication and decreasing the gliding. So it generates stiffness and, at the same time, irritation of the mechanoreceptors within the fascia."

The Stecco team were also the first researchers to understand that the fascia contains nerve endings and therefore can itself be a source of pain, especially when it becomes rigid. As other scientists began to study fascia, these findings were confirmed. In addition, their research helped to show that proprioception (see page 23) is generated through the deep fascia.

Another area the Steccos are currently investigating is the role fascia plays in neuropathy due to nerve entrapment (for instance, in sciatica). "Everybody is focused on the roots of the nerves at the spinal level," Dr. Stecco says, "but in reality, the nerve can be in trouble all the way along." In a recent paper, Dr. Stecco and his colleagues noted that sensory nerves need to cross both the deep and the superficial fascia, creating a significant risk of entrapment if the fascia is very viscous due to microtraumas.[10]

In addition to his work as a researcher, Dr. Stecco teaches classes in Fascial Manipulation®. This method, which involves manipulating the fascia by creating friction over specific points (Centers of Coordination and Centers of Fusion), calls for the practitioner to perform a careful analysis of each individual patient. As a result, Dr. Stecco says, the method produces highly consistent results. He successfully treats wide-ranging problems, not only related to the musculoskeletal system but also including internal dysfunctions such as irritable bowel syndrome, bloating, reflux, dysmenorrhea, incontinence, dysphagia, and more.

Interestingly, Dr. Stecco notes, the points being treated in Fascial Manipulation® are typically not the points where pain occurs. This means the analysis is really about revealing the *source* of the pain—where the fascia is not gliding properly, where the mechanics are off—and treating those points.

Dr. Stecco says that when he treats patients, their strength and range of motion typically improve immediately. "If I were to be honest," he says, "I always expect important results since the first treatment." He also explains that the muscles don't fire completely when there is myofascial dysfunction, which he calls *densification*. Treatment quickly resolves this issue, and the strength in the muscle returns.

Recently, Dr. Stecco's team published exciting research showing that in addition to treating pain, Fascial Manipulation® can have powerful preventive effects.[11] Studying semi-professional soccer players—a group of athletes highly prone to season-ending ankle injuries—the researchers found that performing Fascial Manipulation® on the players at the beginning of the soccer season greatly decreased the number of ankle injuries they experienced over the entire season. "It can restore the mechanics," Dr. Stecco says, "and give a player the best body possible."

CHAPTER 3

YOUR FASCIA: FRIEND OR FOE?

The health of every organ system in your body—in fact, every single cell—depends on your fascia. The health of your fascia, in turn, depends largely on you. Treat your fascia well, and it will be a strong ally. But neglect or mistreat it, and it can become your worst enemy.

So now it's time for you to answer two big questions: (1) How healthy or unhealthy is your fascia? (2) What steps can you take to make your fascia work better for you?

Before you answer these questions, here's one thing you need to know: when it comes to having healthy fascia, no one scores a perfect 10. We all have fascia troubles, whether they stem from injuries, congenital problems, or lifestyle issues. What's more, even the healthiest fascia can become stiff, tight, and dry if it doesn't get a regular workout.

This means that every single one of us can benefit from fascia therapy, even if it's something as simple as massage or foam rolling. It also means that it's smart for us to incorporate lots of stretching and movement into our daily lives. Everything counts, from dancing to practicing yoga to hanging on the monkey bars at the playground.

However, if your fascial problems are serious enough, simple activities like these may not do the trick (and some of them may not be possible for you at this point if you're in pain or have a limited range of motion). That's why my goal in this chapter is to help you decide whether your issues are mild enough to address with do-it-yourself techniques or serious enough that it's time to call on help from professionals.

Using the self-assessment that I've designed, you can evaluate your symptoms and situation and get a good idea about the state of your fascia right now. This knowledge will empower you to plan a course of action that will help you get the strong, flexible, pain-free body you deserve.

Before you begin your self-assessment, however, I'd like to introduce you to four imaginary patients—Sally, Miguel, Lisa, and Jamal—with common fascia problems ranging from small to very serious. These four people are representative of thousands of patients we've seen in our clinic. As you read about their problems and how they solved them, start to think about how similar your own problems and solutions might be.

SMALL PROBLEMS: SALLY

Sally, a 38-year-old single mom and newly promoted HR director for a Silicon Valley tech firm, was getting by—but she knew she could be doing better.

Sally spent eight hours a day slouched in front of her computer. She also sent and received dozens of texts each hour, bending her head down to look at her phone. As a result of her poor posture, she frequently experienced upper back pain, tightness, and myofascial restrictions in her shoulders.

Sally was constantly on the run, juggling her high-stress job with her daughter's busy schedule of piano lessons, soccer, and karate. Although she managed to check off every item on her to-do list each night, she suffered from headaches when the pressure at work and at home—along with the stress of living with a temperamental 15-year-old—got the better of her. Her constant tension caused her to breathe shallowly, making her feel anxious much of the time.

While Sally had a closet full of shoes and boots, she was sad that she couldn't wear many of them anymore because they hurt her feet. As a result, she was forced to switch to flats and tennis shoes.

Sally frequently shorted herself on sleep, and when she finally did get to bed, she tended to toss and turn. In addition, she often grabbed meals on the fly, sacrificing nutrition for convenience.

Despite her stressful life, lack of sleep, bad posture, and poor eating habits, Sally felt okay for the most part. Eventually, however, she decided that simply feeling "okay" wasn't good enough—and that's when she took action.

Sally's Issues and Solutions

Sally's fascia was taking lots of hits each day. Her poor posture and hours of sitting distorted it, her chronic stress constricted it, her poor sleep gave it too little time to rest, and her diet dehydrated it and robbed it of nutrients.

The first step Sally took to turn things around was to begin a yoga class. The breathing and stretching relaxed her fascia, easing the tightness in her back and shoulders. When she combined her yoga with a monthly massage at work, she began to sleep much more soundly, her headaches became fewer and farther between, and she found it easier to cope with her daughter's adolescent moods. Adding in mindful meditation helped her to shake off her stress more easily at the end of the day.

Taking a tip from her yoga instructor, Sally started rolling the fascia at the bottoms of her feet with a tennis ball. Over time, this eased her foot pain, and she could occasionally wear heels again. She also invested in a standing desk (see page 104) so she could switch from sitting to standing for several hours each day. In addition, she started bringing healthy snacks and lunches to work, and she made it a point to stay hydrated. The massage therapist at Sally's office showed her some massage points, and Sally started doing self-massage and foam rolling between her office massages.

Sally's simple steps paid off. Over time, her posture improved, her headaches disappeared, her back and shoulder pain eased, and she had more than enough energy to get through the day.

MODERATE PROBLEMS: MIGUEL

Miguel, a 43-year-old software developer, spent his days at a desk and his nights on the couch surfing the net. He was also a "weekend warrior," pushing himself on long runs to make up for the hours he sat during the week.

Miguel had an old knee injury from playing high school sports. When he ran, his left hip would hurt, the pain extending into his knee. His growing belly and his habit of sitting on his wallet also created hip pain.

A few times a week—especially after his weekend runs—Miguel woke up with a swollen knee or an aching hip. He popped a few ibuprofen each time, and that seemed to quiet things down. However, he worried because his aches and pains bothered him more and more over time. He'd watched his dad become sicker and sicker as he became obese and inactive over the years, and he didn't want to go down the same path.

Miguel's Issues and Solutions

Miguel wanted to do the right thing. However, his habit of sitting too much during the week and then overexercising on the weekends was hurting his fascia, not helping it. His weight gain stressed his fascia as well, and his habit of sitting on his wallet created an imbalance that compressed his fascia on one side and overstretched it on the other.

Miguel's first step was to join a gym, where he received 10 personal training sessions as part of his membership. His personal trainer had him begin a vigorous stretching and stick-rolling routine that Miguel continued doing on his own. The trainer also convinced him to start carrying his wallet in his front pocket. In addition, she used a vibration gun (see page 169) on his painful trigger points.

Miguel also switched from running to swimming, an activity much easier on the fascia in his knees. Resistance training strengthened his weak glutes, a classic problem for runners, helping these muscles to better support his fascia. And rather than limiting his exercise to weekends (and overdoing it then), he started getting off the couch and doing workouts on Tuesdays and Thursdays.

Within months, Miguel's knee and hip pain lessened. His new exercise regimen also helped him to lose five inches off his gut, improving his posture and the health of his fascia.

BIG PROBLEMS: LISA

Lisa, a 36-year-old attorney who hoped to make partner by the age of 40, worked on her computer all day and often long into the night. In addition, she constantly texted clients and fellow attorneys, her neck continuously craned at one screen or another.

While Lisa was slender, she had large breasts. Teased about them in high school, she'd unconsciously developed a slight shoulder hunch to help conceal them. As a result, she suffered from chronic myofascial pain in her neck and upper back, occasionally radiating into her right arm and making her fingers tingle.

Because Lisa worked at a high-powered firm, she dressed in style. She owned a closet full of high heels that looked fabulous but threw her hips and spine out of alignment. She also carried a heavy briefcase, always holding it on her right side, further stressing her neck and back.

Until recently, Lisa had been involved in a serious relationship. However, a year ago, she started experiencing pain during intercourse. She began avoiding sex but was too embarrassed to tell her partner why—especially after her doctor suggested that her problem was psychosomatic. Eventually, her partner became dissatisfied and ended the relationship. She craved companionship, but the idea of dating made her anxious.

Lisa slept only five or six hours a night, relying on a steady supply of sugary coffee drinks to keep her energy up. While this strategy worked temporarily, she woke up feeling tired and stiff each morning and often dragged through her days. She knew that to make partner, she needed to be at the top of her game—and at that point, she wasn't.

Is Pelvic Pain Making You Miserable?

One of the most common and crippling myofascial problems we treat is *chronic pelvic pain*. This pain can strike both men and women, and its effects are often devastating. Symptoms can include the following:

- Pain during or after sex
- Exacerbation of menstrual pain
- Urinary frequency
- Pain when urinating
- Pain when sitting
- Pain in the perineal area (between the vagina and anus or the scrotum and anus)
- Pain during a bowel movement
- Pain in the groin, genitals, coccyx (tailbone), or above the pubic bone
- Lower back pain

In their book *A Headache in the Pelvis*, Drs. David Wise and Rodney Anderson describe pelvic pain as "a vicious cycle of sore pelvic tissue, triggering reflex pelvic muscle tightening, irritating the sore tissue, triggering anxiety, which increases pelvic tension and pain, increasing trigger point electrical activity, and triggering more guarding in the irritated tissue." They compare it to "an ongoing pelvic charley horse."

Pelvic pain can be agonizing. Dr. Anderson, who suffered from it for years before finding relief through what became the Wise-Anderson Protocol, says, "I would wake up in the middle of the night weeping because my pain was so great and I saw no solution." Chronic pelvic pain can also be life-altering, leading to anxiety, depression, isolation, and a loss of interest in sex, and sometimes breaking up relationships.

Despite its severity, doctors often dismiss pelvic pain as solely psychosomatic. Other times, it's misdiagnosed as another medical condition, such as prostatitis or vulvodynia.

> The very good news is that fascia therapy can frequently reduce or even heal chronic pelvic pain, ending years of misery. It may require a combination of approaches; for instance, Drs. Wise and Anderson combine trigger-point therapy and other myofascial release techniques with stress management.

Lisa's Issues and Solutions

Lisa's fascia was constricted due to stress and distorted due to her habit of hunching over. Wearing high heels and carrying her briefcase on one side added to her problems, causing painful fascial restrictions. Her pelvic pain, dismissed as psychosomatic, also stemmed from myofascial issues. The sugary coffee she drank increased her body's production of AGEs (see page 37), which wreak havoc on the sensitive fascia, and her lack of sleep didn't give her fascia enough time to refresh and restore itself.

Luckily, Lisa found answers. A paralegal in her office, hearing about her neck and back pain, recommended a nearby center for integrative medicine. Lisa made an appointment and began a course of care that included physical therapy, chiropractic, acupuncture, massage, and nutritional counseling.

The physical therapist taught Lisa how to stretch the pectoralis muscles in her chest so they could do a better job of supporting her breasts, preventing fascial strictures in her chest area. The therapist also recommended that she save her high heels for special occasions and wear flats or low heels the rest of the time. A physician identified her pelvic pain as myofascial in origin and performed trigger point therapy.

Lisa started alternating between a backpack and a briefcase, and she alternated shoulders when she carried them. She also got an active desk (see page 104) so she could give her fascia a workout even while writing legal briefs. To cope with her stress better, she made deep breathing exercises (see page 65) and mindful meditation (see page 149) part of her daily routine.

Lisa's therapies left her feeling more energized, so she was able to cut down on her sugary coffee. Instead, she made it a habit to drink a fresh green juice every day. She also started getting healthy meals delivered to her office and home so that even when she couldn't cook, she could eat right. As a result, her fascia got the daily doses of water and nutrients it needed.

Lisa is still working crazy hours in a high-stress job. Now, however, she's doing it with more energy and less pain—and she's back on track for the partnership she wants.

SUPERSIZED PROBLEMS: JAMAL

At the age of 45, Jamal had a long history of lower back pain that began when he played on the tennis team in college. In his 20s and early 30s, his back would act up occasionally, but the pain typically resolved after a few days of bed rest. Things went downhill fast, however, when Jamal developed plantar fasciitis, a painful problem affecting the fascia in the bottom of the foot. He tried ice and anti-inflammatories, but they only eased the pain temporarily.

Jamal ended up altering his gait to ease the pain when he walked. As a result, he developed pain in his low back, hip, and knee and had trouble walking. His problems made it harder and harder for him to perform his job as a retail sales manager, which required him to be on his feet all day. His digestion was off a little, too, although he wasn't sure if this was connected to his other issues.

Jamal began using alcohol to help him cope with his pain. He found that a couple of drinks each night would numb him to the point where he could get some sleep.

While Jamal had always been athletic, he had to give up exercising because it hurt too much. As a result, he gained 30 pounds over two years. His blood sugar also began to climb into the prediabetic range—a scary development, since diabetes ran in his family.

Jamal knew that he was at a turning point. He also knew that self-help wouldn't be enough; he needed professional help to take back his life.

Jamal's Issues and Solutions

In Jamal's case, a single crisis—developing plantar fasciitis—triggered a host of secondary problems, ranging from chronic back, hip, and knee pain to digestive issues and, eventually, to alcohol abuse, weight gain, and increased blood sugar. Unfortunately, this downward spiral of pain leading to inactivity, substance abuse, weight gain, and illness is a common story we hear at our clinic. It's a sad tale that many people addicted to opioids or alcohol can tell.

Fortunately, Jamal took action before it was too late. He went to a physiatrist—in other words, a rehab doctor—who drained his knee of inflammation. The physiatrist also gave Jamal some nonsteroidal trigger point injections to break the cycle of fascial pain in his foot and hip.

X-rays revealed that one of Jamal's legs was shorter than the other, impacting his plantar fascia. To correct this problem, the physiatrist prescribed orthotics with a heel lift. Jamal also began an intensive program of physical therapy that included stretching and vibrational treatments to relieve his hip and lower back pain. As an added benefit, this therapy eased his gut problems—not a surprise, since fascial restrictions in the abdomen can cause everything from excess gas to constipation.

In addition, Jamal visited a functional medicine doctor who found that his A1c (a measure of blood sugar levels) was high. In addition to putting him at risk for diabetes, this elevated blood glucose was creating AGEs (see page 37) that damaged his fascia. The doctor put him on a healthy diet and recommended nutritional supplements.

With the help of these interventions, Jamal's pain lessened and eventually disappeared. He was able to stop self-medicating with alcohol and even took up moderate non-weight-bearing exercise to help him get in shape while keeping pressure off his foot. Between his activity and his improved diet, he lost the weight he'd gained. His A1c dropped to 5.3, a normal level—not only lowering his risk for diabetes but also easing the burden on his fascia.

□ □ □

As you can see, there's no "one size fits all" approach to healing the fascia. These four patients had a wide range of symptoms, and they found a variety of solutions to their problems.

Similarly, with a little insight, you can tailor your solutions to meet your own needs. That's why I've designed a simple test to help you evaluate your own fascia and decide your plan of action.

THE "FREE YOUR FASCIA" SELF-ASSESSMENT

Set aside some quiet time to do this test. Give serious thought to each question, and note the pattern of answers for each section.

MEDICAL:

For this section, choose the answers that best describe your health.

Have you ever sprained/strained a joint, torn a ligament, or broken a bone in a way that altered your function?

A. Never
B. A single time
C. Multiple times

Have you experienced any other significant injuries?

A. Never
B. A single time
C. Multiple times

Have you had any surgeries?

A. Never
B. A single surgery
C. Multiple surgeries

Have you experienced emotional trauma or stress for a significant part of your life?

A. Little to no stress
B. Moderate stress
C. Significant stress

What is your body composition?

A. BMI of 18.5–24.9 and/or healthy body fat percentage
B. BMI of 25–29.9 and/or unhealthy body fat percentage
C. BMI of <18.5 or >30 and an unhealthy body fat percentage

Do you have pain anywhere in your body?

A. I'm fully at ease
B. I have a few minor aches and pains
C. I have many regions of minor pain or some regions of moderate to severe pain

Do you have any structural abnormality such as scoliosis, arthritis in a joint, different lengths of limbs, or one shoulder higher than the other?

A. No
B. A minor one that doesn't affect my life
C. Yes, a significant one

Do you have any of the following conditions: fibromyalgia, an inflammatory disease, temporomandibular joint disorder, diabetes or prediabetes, or migraines?

A. No
B. No, but it runs in my family
C. Yes

How is your blood pressure?

A. Within normal range
B. Slightly out of normal range, but managed without medication
C. High

How is your range of motion?

A. I move with ease
B. I have no major restrictions, but I could be more flexible
C. I have a restricted range of motion (with or without pain) and it significantly interferes with my everyday activities

What is your balance like?

A. I move with grace and ease
B. Normal, but could be improved
C. I am clumsy, trip easily, and/or have poor balance

Do you experience urinary leakage when you cough, sneeze, laugh, or exercise?

A. No
B. No, but this was a past concern/is likely to become a future concern
C. Yes

Is pain or limited range of motion interfering with your sex life?

A. No
B. No, but this was a past concern/is likely to become a future concern
C. Yes

LIFESTYLE:

For this section, choose the answers that you relate to more.

Do you drink water throughout the day?

A. I make a conscious effort to drink water every day
B. I often forget to drink water

What is your usual diet like?

A. I eat a high-nutrient diet rich in fruits and vegetables, low in processed food
B. I occasionally eat processed food

Do you avoid sugar?

A. I read labels and avoid products with added sugar
B. Sugary treats are a normal part of my diet

How much sleep do you usually get each night?

A. More than seven hours
B. Less than seven hours

Do you take a nutritional supplement?

A. I regularly take a full-spectrum supplement
B. I take no supplements or often forget to take them

How much activity do you regularly get each day (include workouts, housework, yard work, etc.)?

A. At least 60 minutes of moderate to intense activity every day
B. Less than 60 minutes daily or only light activity

Do you frequently vary your exercise?

A. I often try new activities or work different muscle groups
B. I like routine and doing the same exercises

How often do you stretch each week?

A. More than 10 minutes a day, at least three days a week
B. Rarely to never

How often do you get bodywork (e.g., massage or acupuncture)?

A. At least monthly
B. Never to rarely

Do you practice stress-reducing activities (e.g., yoga or meditation)?

A. Regularly
B. Never to rarely

Do you cumulatively sit for more than 8 hours each day (include work, home, and driving time)?

A. No, I am usually on my feet
B. Yes, but I try to stand up every hour or two
C. Yes, and I'm often stuck sitting for hours without a break

How do you hold your phone when you send or read text messages?

A. I rarely look at my phone and/or consciously practice good posture while sending and receiving texts
B. I'm not mindful of my posture, but I'm on my phone for less than an hour a day
C. I'm craned over my phone all day

Do you often bend your neck to use your shoulder to hold your phone to your ear?

A. No
B. Yes, for occasional long phone sessions
C. Yes, I'm regularly on my phone and usually bending my neck to keep it in place

How often do you play video games?

A. Occasionally or never
B. More than 10 hours a week, including marathon sessions

Do you wear high heels?

A. Never or only for special occasions
B. Yes, at least three times a week

How heavy is your regular bag?

A. I carry no bag or a light bag that is easy to lift
B. Heavy enough to feel it in my muscles when I set it down

If you have an everyday bag, how do you usually carry it?

A. I regularly switch the arm or shoulder I carry my bag on
B. I usually carry my bag on the same side

Do you regularly put things in your back pocket?

A. No—if I do, I remove them before sitting
B. Yes, I often keep bulky things, like my phone or wallet, in a back pocket

Where do you usually place your legs and feet when you sit?

A. Feet planted on the floor—when I cross my legs, I alternate the top leg
B. Legs crossed, with the same leg on top

Does your daily life require you to make the same repetitive motions each day (e.g., typing or caring for a baby)?

A. No
B. Yes
C. Yes, and I have stress injuries due to this activity

Do you feel you are under a great deal of stress?

A. No
B. Sometimes
C. Regularly

Do you smoke?

A. No, never
B. Sometimes (or previously)
C. Regularly

What is your alcohol consumption in an average week?

A. None
B. Moderate (up to 7 drinks for women, up to 14 for men)
C. Heavy (7+ drinks for women, 14+ for men; more than 3–4 drinks at any sitting)

When you exercise, what do you do when you encounter pain?

A. Ease the intensity, perhaps pause to recheck form
B. Push through it—no pain, no gain!

SELF-REFLECTION:

For this section, give yourself an A if you do relate to the sentence; B if you do not.

I have lots of energy and a spring in my step.

I am strong.

I am graceful.

I am flexible.

I have good posture.

I am aging well.

I am physically able to do everyday tasks with ease.

I am at peace with myself and the world.

TO SCORE:

If you answered C to any question at all, or if you have any medical problems not addressed here that significantly impact your health, you owe it to yourself to obtain a professional evaluation. I recommend going to a holistic clinic that can address your issues from multiple angles. You are extremely likely to have a significant fascia problem, and while self-help measures can be beneficial, they may not be sufficient.

Now, look at your pattern of B answers:

- If you have B answers in the medical section, it's a smart idea to have at least one consultation with a professional. However, there's a good chance that you can optimize your fascia largely through self-therapy, including lifestyle changes and exercise.

- If you have B answers in the lifestyle section, you can address every one of these issues with simple lifestyle changes, self-therapy, and an occasional bodywork session (for instance, a massage).

- If you have B answers in the self-reflection section, I recommend starting with self-help and with simple professional therapies such as massage, and then graduating to professional help if these measures don't adequately address your problem areas.

These guidelines are a good starting point. However, you're in charge of your fascia therapy, so choose what works best for you, your lifestyle, and your budget. There are dozens and dozens of different types of fascia therapy, and there's no right or wrong approach. They all work, because they all address the fascia. If you address your fascia in some way, shape, or form, you will make progress.

PART II

THE "FREE YOUR FASCIA" PROGRAM

Whether you opt for do-it-yourself therapies or seek professional help, you'll have lots of fascia-oriented therapies to choose from. While the list is growing every year, here's a sampling of the many names you'll hear when you search out therapies that focus on fascia:

- Rolling
- Dynamic (Active) and Static Stretching
- John F. Barnes Myofascial Release Approach
- Stretch to Win
- Rolfing (Structured Integration)
- The Melt Method (created by Sue Hitzmann)
- Fascial Fitness
- Myofascial Trigger Point Therapy (Janet G. Travell method)
- Visceral Manipulation
- Fascial Manipulation (Stecco method)
- Active Release Technique (ART)
- The Graston Technique
- Feldenkrais

- The Stick
- Gyrotonic
- Alexander technique
- Yoga
- Pilates
- Tai Chi

- Massage
- Acupuncture/ Acupressure
- Vibration
- Trigger Point Injections
- Hydration (Quench)

While there are many different "flavors" of fascia therapy, they fall into basic categories including stretching, rolling, vibration, posture-enhancing exercises, acupuncture/acupressure, trigger point therapy, orthotics, and lifestyle changes. In the self-help chapters that follow, I'll introduce you to methods you can do on your own, using inexpensive equipment or no equipment at all. After that, I'll tell you about powerful tools that professionals can offer you.

No matter which route you choose, here is the most important thing: get started! Each step you take to free your fascia, large or small, will bring you closer to having a healthy, strong, and flexible body—and that's an exciting journey to begin.

A Note for Athletes

For the most part, athletes aren't that different from anyone else when it comes to fascial injuries or restrictions. But here's where they *are* very different: rather than simply going for feeling good, they're going for gold. As a result, most will go above and beyond to gain even the slightest edge in competition.

If this sounds like you, then you definitely want to have fascia experts on your training team. Optimizing your fascia can do everything from increasing your range of motion to helping you prevent injuries. In addition, addressing fascial constrictions in your ribcage can increase your ability to breathe deeply and oxygenate your blood. I strongly recommend reading *Fascia in Sport and Movement*, edited by Robert Schleip, Ph.D., for in-depth information about fascia therapies for athletes.

CHAPTER 4

RELEASE YOUR FASCIA BY STRETCHING

Cats, dogs, and people all love a good stretch first thing in the morning. That stretch feels wonderful because it loosens, hydrates, and lubricates fascia that gets stiff, tight, and sticky after a night's sleep. (Yawning when you first wake up is also a great way to hydrate the fascia in your face and neck.)

However, your fascia needs much more than a single morning stretch to satisfy its craving for movement. To keep it fluid and free from knots and restrictions, you need to commit to a daily stretching and/or movement routine that involves *every part of your body* from head to toe.

Stretching every day is especially important if you have chronic pain. I know that pain tends to make you want to move less, and it can be difficult to overcome that instinct. But daily stretching in the correct ways can ease pain—often dramatically—and it often reduces the need for pain medications. Here's a sampling of research findings that support stretching for pain:

- In one study, researchers randomly divided 102 patients with acute plantar fasciitis pain into two groups. One group stretched three times a day for eight weeks, and the other underwent standard shockwave therapy. Following up on the patients, the researchers found that 65 percent of patients who did the stretches reported total or nearly total satisfaction with the outcome, compared to a 29 percent satisfaction rate in the shockwave therapy group.[1]

- In a separate experiment, 96 office workers with moderate to severe neck pain received a brochure about proper posture and ergonomics. Researchers then instructed half the group to perform neck and shoulder stretches twice a day, five days a week, for four weeks. The office workers doing the exercises had significantly decreased pain, improved neck function, and increased quality of life compared to the control group who received the brochure alone. Furthermore, the office workers who did the exercises at least three times per week had even greater function and higher quality-of-life scores than those who did them less often.[2]

- Other studies show that stretching can decrease pain after a hamstring injury, reduce pain and increase function in patients with shoulder pain, increase range of motion and decrease pain in women with muscular skeletal symptoms, and minimize lower back pain and disability.[3]

So, stretching can work wonders when it comes to pain relief—and better yet, a stretching routine that keeps your fascia in peak form can help to prevent pain in the first place. The trick is to stretch regularly and to do it the right way.

TWO RIGHT WAYS (AND ONE WRONG WAY) TO STRETCH

There are two types of stretching you can use to elongate, hydrate, and lubricate your fascia: *active* stretching (also called *dynamic* stretching) and *static* stretching.

In active stretching, you move through your full range of motion, but you don't hold a stretch for more than a few seconds at the end. Examples include arm circles, leg swings, waist twists, and butt kicks. In static stretching—for instance, traditional hamstring stretches—you hold the stretch for a longer time, typically 20 to 90 seconds.

In each type of stretching, your goal is to move through your full range of motion. You want to move just to the point of discomfort, but not beyond. Over time, the point of discomfort should be farther and deeper into the stretch.

In this chapter, I'll share my favorite stretches for relaxing and hydrating the fascia. (In Chapter 5, you'll find additional stretches and other exercises designed specifically to improve your posture.) I recommend stretching daily, focusing in particular on tight areas.

Note on ballistic stretching: Ballistic stretches are stretches with a bounce at the end. One example is bouncing as you try to touch your toes. Unlike static or active (dynamic) stretching, ballistic stretching forces you to move outside of your safe range of motion. Because of this, it carries a fairly high risk for injury, and I don't recommend it.

THE GROUND RULES FOR STRETCHING

To stretch safely, and to get the most benefit from your stretches, follow these rules:

- Although your first stretch in the morning feels great, wait for at least an hour after getting out of bed to do your actual stretching regimen. Your body will be less stiff, and more ready for some serious stretching, after you've moved around a bit.

- Always breathe deeply and consistently while stretching (more on this shortly). Many people have a tendency to hold their breath if a stretch is painful—which makes it more painful!—but breathing during stretching oxygenates your blood, increases your circulation, and helps to clean out toxins.

- If one area of your body feels particularly tight or painful, try starting with that area first. This may open up other areas if you are guarding them. (However, avoid stretching areas that are still healing from an acute injury.) Interestingly, the opposite may also occur: if you stretch the areas around a particularly tight or painful spot, you may open it up. See which method works best for you.

- Stretch your body in as many directions as possible, and try lots of different ways of moving. Experiment— be your own petri dish! Be conscious of what does and doesn't work for you.

- After you stretch, rest and drink water. This will allow your body to pump new water back into your fascia after you've pumped stale water out.

- Watch for asymmetries. For instance, you may notice that your right side is more restricted than your left side when you do a stretch. When you detect an asymmetry, double the number of repetitions you do on the restricted side. If you don't notice a change over time, you may have an underlying issue that requires professional help.

- Add icing or heating to your regimen if you want to make your stretches even more productive. (See more on this on page 67.)

- If you're combining your stretches with a workout, do dynamic stretches before you exercise to activate your fascia and muscles. However, avoid doing static stretches before you work out, because research shows that these can actually lower your performance.[4] Instead, do static stretches *after* you exercise, when your muscles are warm and fatigued and more primed to stretch.

Important: Breathe as You Stretch!

To get the most benefit from your stretches, you need to breathe deeply and regularly throughout them. If you're not used to deep breathing, practice it until it becomes a habit. Here's how to do it:

- Placing your thumbs at the lower edge of your ribs, spread the rest of your fingers over your belly. Relax your shoulders and face.

- Breathe in through your nose and out through your mouth, feeling the movement under your hands.

- As you inhale, consciously fill your belly with air like a balloon. Then, as you breathe out, pull your belly in toward your spine.

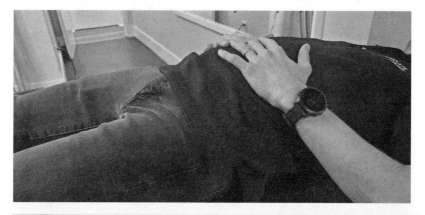

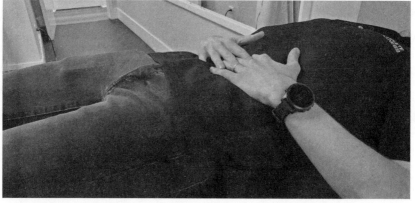

Expanding and contracting your belly as you breathe.

- Next, lengthen your exhalation so it's longer than your inhalation. This will enhance your relaxation.
- Occasionally, breathe faster for a minute or two. (This helps to build strength.)

As you're stretching, consciously monitor your breathing. Eventually, deep breathing will become a habit.

HOW STRETCHING PAYS OFF

Stretching is an easy habit to get into because you can do it anywhere and anytime—at home, at your desk, on your lunch break. You can also multitask by stretching while you're watching a movie, listening to music, or talking on the phone. (I do stretches while in the elevator of my high-rise apartment building.) It takes only a few minutes each day to stretch your fascia, and you'll reap the benefits all day and night:

- Increased flexibility and range of motion
- Reduced pain
- Improved symmetry
- Better athletic performance
- Reduced risk of injury
- Improved energy
- Improved circulation
- Decreased stress
- Increased mobility
- Improved balance
- Better sleep

In short, while stretching is simple, it's powerful medicine for your myofascial system. (That's one reason why every culture in the world instinctively gravitates toward activities that stretch the fascia—from tai chi to salsa dancing to Twister.) Make daily stretching part of your lifestyle, and you'll be amazed at the physical and mental benefits you see.

ICE AND HEAT WITH STRETCHING

Many people like to add ice or heat to their regimen to make their stretches more productive. Especially when it comes to fascial injuries, there are many strong opinions on the virtues of either method. Chiropractor Dr. Sabrina Atkins says: "The one rule I have in terms of heat and ice is it's 10 minutes max for either one of them. I limit ice because I want to encourage blood flow, and I limit heat because of the potential to slow healing. I want to calm the tissue a little bit, but I don't want to impact its ability to heal. Often, I don't use ice or heat at all. I focus more on creating blood flow and healing activity through active movement and conscious awareness."

To know whether adding ice or heat is best for you, I recommend experimenting by limiting your use to 10 minutes for each method. Then pause and feel which is more productive and helps your stretching in the short term as well as the long term.

Brent Anderson, Ph.D.: "Fascia Is Part of Everything"

Brent Anderson, Ph.D., is the co-creator of Polestar Pilates, one of the world's leading Pilates education authorities. He is a licensed physical therapist and orthopedic certified specialist with more than two decades of experience.

How does your approach affect the fascia?

When load is placed on fascia, it changes its shape and orientation. The Pilates environment is a beautiful environment that allows us to manipulate load. What I'm playing with in my Pilates environment is *manipulation of load and gravity.*

For instance, I can take a leg that feels very heavy to somebody who just had a hip replacement or has an inguinal hernia or sciatica pain, and I can suspend that leg and take off 50 percent of the load. In this way, I can create an appropriate amount of load for a sustained period of time in a dynamic load setting.

If I want to create a structural change, and I want that structural change to carry over into functional movements, but the person isn't prepared to handle a full load of gravity, I can use the Pilates equipment to create a dynamic load environment that will educate the fascia: "This is how you should sustain yourself. Your purpose is to be able to maintain these ranges of motions and these load-bearing movements."

When someone finishes the treatment, and I say, "How do you feel?" they say, "Oh, I feel lighter. I feel grounded in my feet. I feel more space. I feel more warmth and flow and energy." That's because, when the skeleton is aligned in its optimal position, there's less load on the elastic chains of the fascial system.

Like me, you work with many people who sit all day long. How much damage does too much sitting do?

I can't remember who originally said it, but the fascia is like a 3-D printer. When we put ourselves in a position, our fascia is just printing the position we're in. So if we're always sitting, then our fascia looks like sitting fascia. There isn't elasticity in the posterior chain.

When we ask people who sit all day to do a good exercise for glutes, they feel it in their quads instead. They don't ever feel it in their glutes, no matter how we try to position it. It's like the chain has been shut off. Their knees collapse in, their feet collapse down, they have flat feet, they have bunions. You see this whole pattern of poor myofascial organization in relationship to vertical posture. It all collapses. This is why it's important to motivate people who have sedentary lifestyles to become more active, and to encourage people with poor posture to improve their posture.

Many people with chronic pain think that bodywork can't help them because their physical limitations are too severe. However, your own research is encouraging in this regard. Can you talk a little about that?

My doctoral dissertation looked at the psychosocial impact of successful movement experiences in people with chronic back pain.

We know that physical limitations—for instance, range of motion, strength, power, core strength, flexibility, coordination—are very poor predictors of outcome in back pain. All of these measures at best have something like a 50 percent correlation to functional outcomes.

What we actually found when people with low back pain did Pilates was that *simply having successful movement experiences*—that is, experiences that did not cause pain or fear—changed how they perceived their well-being. And that correlated very strongly with whether or not people got better.

FASCIA, STRETCHING, AND CANCER: WHAT WE DO AND DON'T KNOW

Stretching can do everything from easing pain to making us more flexible—but could it even reduce our risk of getting cancer? Recently, Helene Langevin and her colleagues conducted an experiment to find out.

Langevin and colleagues stretched mice by holding them by the tail and gently lifting them, allowing their front paws to grasp a bar. They then compared the mice who stretched for several minutes each day with a "no stretch" group.

The researchers injected the mammary tissue of mice in both groups with breast cancer cells. They found that after four weeks, tumor volume was 52 percent smaller in the mice that stretched compared to the controls.

Hypothesizing that stretching may rev up cancer-fighting T cells, the team measured the levels of molecular markers that signal the activation of an immune response. They found that stretching reduced levels of PD-1, a key immune "checkpoint" that blocks the body's ability to fight cancer cells. The team also measured levels of specialized pro-resolving mediators (SPMs), which are molecules that help to resolve inflammation. They found that levels of SPMs were significantly greater in the stretch group than in the control group.

The researchers concluded, "Stretching is a gentle, non-pharmacological intervention that could become an important component of cancer treatment and prevention."

Commenting on the research, Langevin said, "Inflammation is a double-edged sword in cancer. Although it is an essential component of all immune responses, it needs to be limited both in location and duration. Finding changes in both markers of the immune system ramping up its attack on cancer cells as well as markers of inflammation resolution suggests a potentially important link between these two areas of inquiry."[5]

While the research is intriguing, it's in its early stages, so it's too soon to tell if stretching truly can reduce the risk of some types of cancer. Also, researchers don't yet know if stretching after a cancer diagnosis could decrease or increase the spread of the disease. (There is concern that when cancerous cells are already present, stretching might increase the likelihood of metastatic "seeding.") These are yet more fascia mysteries remaining to be solved.

In the meantime, however, I've heard some very exciting anecdotes from fellow practitioners. For instance, I recently talked with Aaron Mattes, who is a pioneer in fascia therapy, the inventor of a technique called Active Isolated Stretching (AIS), and one of my good friends and mentors. During our conversation, he told me about two remarkable cases from his own practice.

The first case, he says, involved a woman with a cancerous brain tumor the size of a grapefruit who was undergoing chemotherapy and radiation therapy. Following four treatments by Mattes, scans showed that the tumor had shrunk to the size of an acorn—and after two more treatments, it had disappeared. Her oncologist commented that in 35 years of practice, he had never seen the mass of a tumor like hers change.

The second case involved a woman with stage iv breast cancer who was given less than a month to live. After several rounds of AIS, she had a blood test. "What do you think they found?" Mattes asked me. "Her cancer had totally disappeared. And four years later, she's still alive."

Right now, the jury is out on whether myofascial work will become a powerful tool in our cancer-fighting arsenal. Time (and much more scientific research) will tell—but so far, the laboratory studies and anecdotal reports are highly encouraging.

NINE GREAT STRETCHES FOR YOUR FASCIA

These stretches will work every major area of your body in just a few minutes. Do extra repetitions to stretch any area that feels especially tight. Always stretch to the point of pain, never beyond. Also, remember to continue slow, relaxed breathing as you stretch.

If you have significant fascial or medical issues that affect your ability to stretch, or you're short on time, start with two or three stretches each day, focusing on the areas that bother you most. Starting with the biggest muscle groups, such as your hamstrings, is best.

If stretching is difficult for you at first, begin with only one or two repetitions, and gradually increase the number of repetitions you do. Add new stretches as you get stronger, but avoid any stretches that are too difficult for you.

If you are able to do more, try to do most or all of the stretches every day. Once you've learned how to do each stretch, the entire series should only take you about 12 to 15 minutes total.

To get even more benefit from your stretches, combine them with affirmations (see Chapter 7). For instance, as you stretch, you can say one of the following to yourself:

- "I am strong and flexible."

- "My stretching empowers me to live a pain-free life."

- "My fascia is free and liquid."

- "The more I stretch, the more supple and relaxed I become."

Note: For a few of these exercises, you will need a yoga strap or looped stretching strap (see photo that follows for examples) or a belt or bathrobe tie.

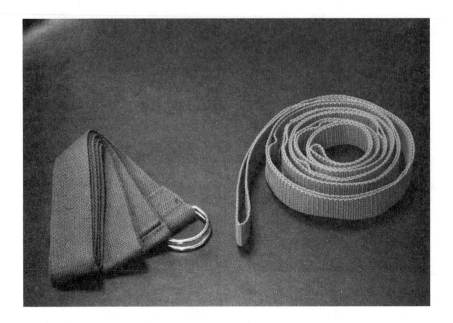

Stretch 1: Plantar Fascia Stretch

This is an excellent exercise if you've been diagnosed with plantar fasciitis or if you have pain in the plantar fascia (a thick band of fascia that runs along the bottom of your foot from your heel to your toes) when you first get up in the morning.

However, even if the bottom of your foot is not a problem, do this stretch daily. The bottom of your foot is where your kinetic chain (see Chapter 1) begins, and looser is better. Restrictions can translate into pain in other areas of the body, so this is a great preventive. If I were going to recommend one stretch for people with no issues, I would tell them to stretch their feet.

To do this exercise, you'll need a yoga strap, belt, or bathrobe tie. Make a loop in the strap, belt, or tie and place the loop around the ball of your foot, holding the other end of the strap, belt, or tie with one hand. Point your toes down, then pull them up toward your head. Go back and forth 20 times each session, 10 to 12 times a day.

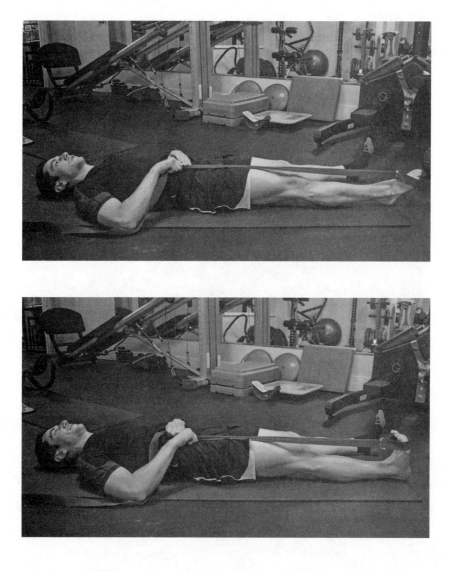

Stretch 2: Low Back Side Stretch

This exercise will help to correct an imbalance in the strength of your back muscles, which in turn will help to correct or prevent fascial restrictions.

Stand with your feet shoulder width apart. Place your right middle finger on the right side of your thigh and slide it down your leg as you bend to the right, contracting the muscles in the right side of your lower back. Be careful not to twist your body forward or backward. (If you're wearing pants with a side seam, slide down the seam.) Do 8 to 10 repetitions, and then repeat on the other side.

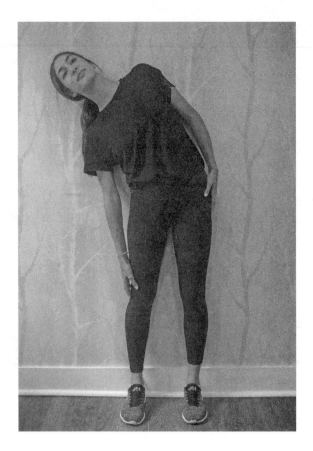

Stretch 3: Cobra Yoga Pose

This classic yoga position will help to release the fascia in the front of your torso and a muscle called the psoas (more on the psoas shortly) that's very important for good posture and gait. It's an essential stretch for those who sit.

Start on your stomach with your legs straight behind you and your chin touching the floor. Bend your elbows, and place your palms on the floor, as close to your body as possible. Take a deep breath in, and on the exhale, push up with your hands while pushing your pelvis into the floor. Concentrate on using your back muscles to lift your upper body. Hold this position for 10 seconds, and then lower yourself back to the floor. Repeat 8 to 10 times.

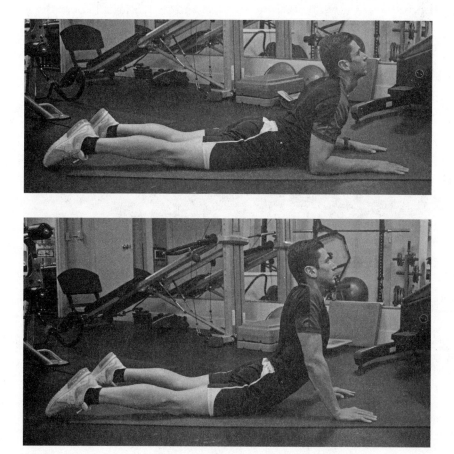

Stretch 4: Psoas Series

The psoas muscles flex your hips and help to stabilize and support your lower back. These are some of the most important muscles for steady upright standing and walking. Stretching them can improve your alignment and protect against fascial restrictions in your back and hips.

For the first part of this exercise, lie on a bed with your lower legs hanging down. Lift your right leg with your knee bent, and hold it up with your hands on the front of your shin, just below your knee, as shown. Straighten your left leg, pulling your foot down so you feel the stretch in the front of your hip. Be sure to keep your left knee straight and your left foot off the floor. Hold for 30 to 90 seconds. Return to your starting position and switch legs. Repeat three to four times on each leg.

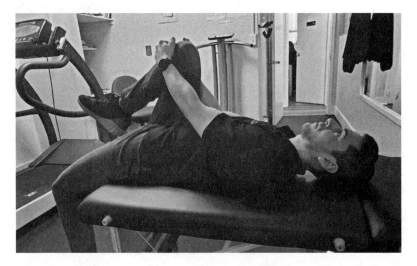

For the second part of this exercise, remain on the bed. Keep your right leg down and pull your left knee up toward your head, hands behind your left thigh. Point your left toes away from your head, then point your toes toward your head, pushing your left heel away from your body by pushing your left hip down. (Visualize your waistline dropping on your left side.) Hold for 30 to 90 seconds. Do 3 to 4 repetitions on each side.

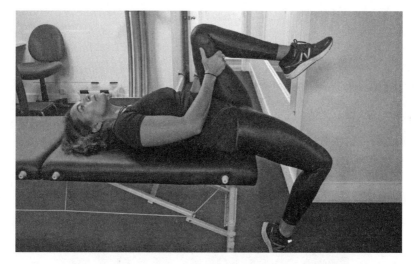

For the third part of this exercise, kneel on the ground. Your right knee should touch the floor, your left leg bent in front of you so your left foot is flat on the ground. Raise your right hand toward the ceiling and then bend your torso all the way to the left. Do four or five 20-second repetitions and then repeat on the other side.

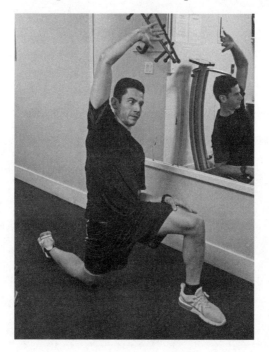

Stretch 5: Three-Part Neck Stretch

This stretch focuses on three different sets of neck muscles: the muscles at the front, side, and back.

First, use the muscles of your neck to tilt your head to the right side. Then, with your right hand on top of your head, pull your head farther to the right. Hold for a long count of one, then go back to the center. Do 10 stretches, and then repeat on the other side.

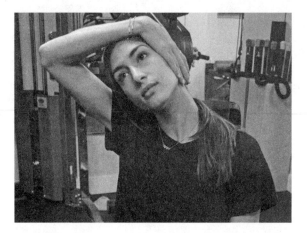

Now turn your head 45 degrees to the right and tilt it slightly backward. Then place your right hand on the top of your head, and gently pull on your head to increase the tilt. Be sure your torso stays still so your neck is doing the work. Your head is the only thing that should move. Do 10 stretches, and then repeat on the other side.

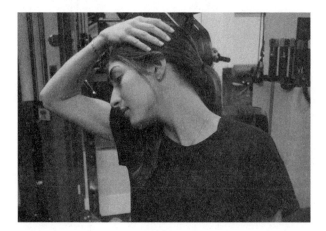

Now, holding your head at the same 45-degree angle, move your head forward using the muscles of the neck. Then place your right hand on top of your head, and gently pull your head farther forward, pushing your ear toward your right armpit. Again, be sure your torso stays still. You should feel the pulling from the base of your skull right into your shoulder blade. Do 10 repetitions, and repeat on the left side.

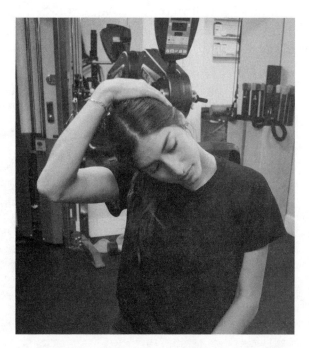

Stretch 6: Cat Curl Yoga

This stretch works wonders for the fascia in your back and core.

Start on your hands and knees, with your back straight. Taking a deep breath in, bring your back into an upside-down "U" shape by lifting your abdominal muscles, tucking your pelvis in, and pushing your nose toward your pelvis. Now, breathe out as you bring your spine into a right-side-up "U" by dropping your abdominal muscles, lifting your buttocks, and lifting your head in the direction of your buttocks. Keep your arms straight and stable so your body does not rock forward or back.

Note: If you find this stretch challenging, you can do a "half cat curl." To do this, simply do either the first or second part of the exercise—not both—and then return to a neutral position.

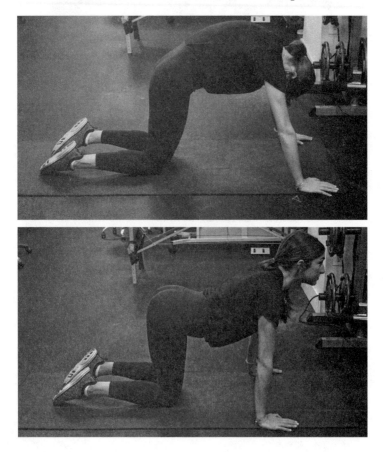

Stretch 7: Hip Stretch Series

This five-part stretch will give the fascia in your hip a good work-out. Do five repetitions on each side. Be sure not to bend your spine during these stretches; the motion should originate from your hip.

First, lie on the floor. Using a yoga strap or belt, make a loop, and wrap it around the ball of your right foot. Now, holding the strap or belt in your hands, lift your right leg straight up in the air, giving it a gentle pull toward you at the top of the motion. Repeat on the opposite side.

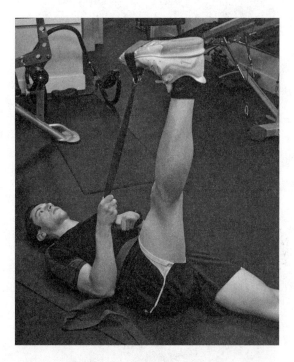

This time, again using the strap or belt, lift your right leg and pull it toward your left shoulder. Use one or both hands on the strap or belt to guide your leg. Again, give the leg a gentle pull at the top of the motion. Repeat on the opposite side.

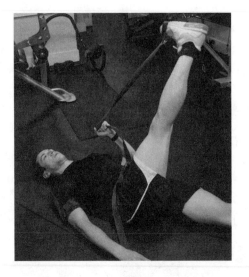

Now, holding the strap in your left hand, move your right leg toward the left side of your body at a 45-degree angle from the floor. Again, give the leg a gentle pull at the top of the motion. Repeat on the opposite side.

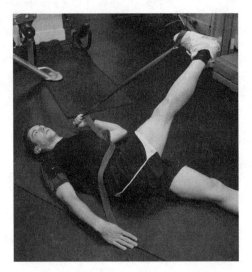

Next, holding the band in your left hand, lift your right leg straight up; then, moving your left arm out from your body, pull your right leg toward the left side of your body. Again, give the leg a gentle pull at the end of the motion. Repeat on the opposite side.

For the final stretch, you will not need the yoga strap. Lying on your back, bend your right knee. Now move the knee toward the opposite shoulder. Grabbing the knee with both hands, pull it gently toward the shoulder. Repeat on the opposite side.

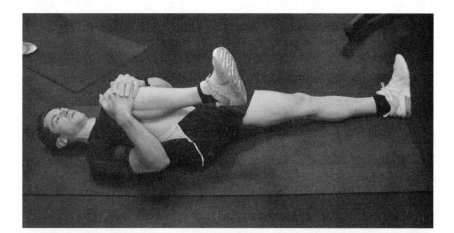

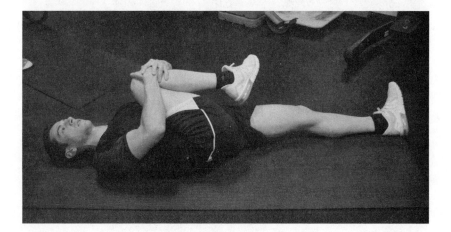

Stretch 8: Erect Sitting Tall Head Posture

When you sit, you have a tendency to let your head jut forward. When you sit a lot, your myofascia contracts and adapts to that position.

This exercise is meant to stretch the myofascia to help reshape it, as well as to strengthen the muscles of the back of the neck to prevent that jutting forward. This is a great exercise to do in front of your computer; after you're done, try to maintain the tall posture when you resume your work.

Begin by sitting with your back off the chair and your butt as far forward as possible, which will roll your pelvis forward. Your feet should be flat on the floor. Your knees should be directly in front of your hips, not flared out, and should be bent at a 90-degree angle. Your hands should be relaxed and placed on your thighs.

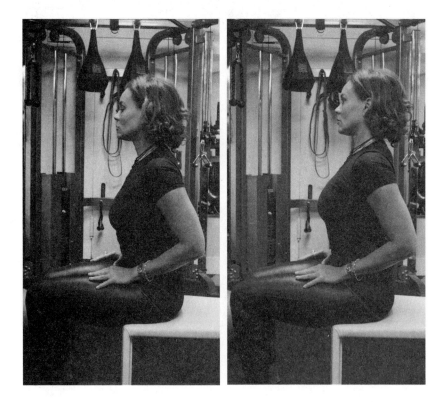

Sit as tall as possible, with your abdominal muscles engaged—remember to breathe! (Use the belly breathing that you learned on page 65.)

Once you're in position, do this:

Part 1: Glide your head backward on your spine. It's important that you simply glide gently here. Gliding backward will make your chest puff out, which is fine. The goal of Part 1 is to have your head in back of your torso.

Part 2: From the backward glided position, tilt your head 10 or 15 degrees upward (looking skyward) by contracting the muscles of the back of the neck. Hold for 15 to 20 seconds. Repeat 10 times.

Stretch 9: The Doorway Stretch

This exercise will stretch the muscles and fascia of your chest and shoulders. In addition, it will help you build and maintain core strength.

Stand in a doorway and place your hands on either side of the doorframe at a comfortable height at or above shoulder level. Take an approximately six-inch step backward out of the doorway to reduce strain on your chest and upper back. Your feet should be shoulder width apart. Engage your abs, and keep your head and chest lifted. Now take a deep breath. As you exhale, lean against your hands, making sure you do not let your pelvis come forward. You could think of this as a Standing Plank.

Breathe naturally, and hold the stretch for a count of 20. Over time, increase the count to 60 seconds.

After the Doorway Stretch, you will feel open in your chest.

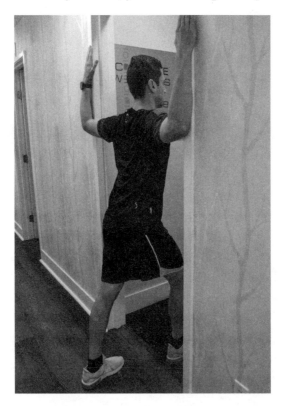

WHAT TO EXPECT WHEN YOU STRETCH

If you're like most people, I predict that you'll feel a difference even after your first day of stretching. You may feel more balanced, lighter on your feet, even a little taller. Your movements will be looser and freer. You may also get a little hit of happiness—an added bonus—because stretching releases the feel-good neurotransmitter dopamine.

Keep up your stretching, and you'll continue to see changes. As you free your fascia, you'll relieve pain in areas that are now tight and restricted. You'll become more flexible. You'll develop better balance. If you're into sports, your performance will get better. You'll have more energy, feel better, and even sleep better.

So make stretching a daily habit for the rest of your life. Your fascia will thank you!

CHAPTER 5

OPTIMIZE YOUR FASCIA BY STANDING TALL

The next time you're out in public, look at the people around you. How many are hunching their shoulders, holding their heads too far forward (we call it "turtle neck"), or walking or standing in an awkward way? How many people, on the other hand, are sitting, standing, and walking with beautiful posture?

Now, guess which people have free, healthy fascia. Yes—it's the group with gorgeous posture.

Ida Rolf, a famous early pioneer in fascia therapy, once said, "Fascia is the organ of posture." This might surprise you if you think that it's your muscles and bones that hold you upright. Of course, both muscles and bones do play a role in your posture—but without your fascia creating structure via the tensegrity we talked about in Chapter 1, you would simply collapse into a heap.

So when you think of your posture, don't just think about your bones and muscles—think about your fascia as well. When your fascia is free, you can stand strong and tall. When it's brittle and bound, you can't.

THE CONNECTION BETWEEN POSTURE AND FASCIA, MOOD, AND MORE

Just as healthy fascia promotes good posture, good posture promotes healthy fascia. The fascia-posture connection is a two-way street. If you have good posture, you can sit and stand and move correctly. This helps to prevent kinks and knots from developing in your fascia, so it can glide with ease. Conversely, if you have bad posture, you sit, stand, and move in ways that compress or over-stretch your fascia, distorting and binding it.

The way you hold yourself while standing, sitting, and walking has an impact on other areas of your life as well, such as your mood, energy levels, and stress levels. Over time, bad physical posture turns into bad "mental posture." To experience this yourself, stand up straight with your head high and your shoulders strong. Then hunch your back and shoulders and let your head drop. Did you feel the immediate change in your mood, from confident and happy to negative and self-limiting?

Research confirms that posture affects mood. In one study, psychologists found that walking in a slouched posture decreases energy and increases negative emotions such as sadness, loneliness, isolation, and sleepiness. When slouching, study participants reported feeling "zombie-like" or "wanting to just sit down." By contrast, when they stood upright while skipping and swinging their arms in opposition to their legs, they reported higher levels of energy and positive feelings like happiness.[1]

Good posture can also help you breathe easier. In a separate study, researchers administered breathing tests to 15 young men. In one condition, the men sat upright. In the other, they sat hunched over with their heads forward. (If you text all day on a smartphone, this is what you're doing.) The result: in the hunched position, the men's respiratory function immediately and dramatically got worse.

Next, the researchers asked participants to rotate their heads to one side and flex their sides to the other, a posture similar to that seen in a condition called *torticollis*. This is a position frequently associated with neck muscle spasms. Again, the effects on the participants' breathing were immediate and negative.[2]

In another study, researchers asked people to participate in two stressful activities (giving a speech and counting backward in steps of 13) while sitting in a slouched or upright position. The researchers reported, "Upright participants reported higher self-esteem, more arousal, better mood, and lower fear, compared to slumped participants." In addition, the study showed that "slumped partici-pants used more negative emotion words, first-person singular pro-nouns, affective process words, sadness words, and fewer positive emotion words and total words during the speech." The researchers commented, "Sitting upright may be a simple behavioral strategy to help build resilience to stress."[3]

BEGIN BY ANALYZING YOUR POSTURE

One of the best ways to free your fascia is to create and maintain good posture. In this chapter, I'll share simple exercises that will empower you to do this. First, however, I'd like to give you a little insight into how good (or not-so-good) your posture is right now. To do this, I'd like you to do two quick self-analyses.

The Mirror Exercise

Do this exercise in front of a full-length mirror. Standing in front of the mirror, close your eyes and gently shake the tension out of every part of your body: your arms, legs, shoulders, hips, and head (avoid straining or jerking your neck). Even do a couple of easy jumps, being careful not to lose your balance and fall. When you open your eyes, try not to correct your posture. We want you to see the real you, the posture you use on a daily basis.

Now start your assessment from the bottom up. Take notice of the following:

- Are your feet parallel, or is one foot in front of the other?

- Is there more weight in your heels or your toes, or is your weight even and centered?

- Is there more weight on your right foot or left foot, or is your weight equal on both sides?

- Is one of your feet turned out or turned in more than the other?

- Is one of your legs more turned out compared to the other?

- Are your knees buckled in, buckled out, or facing forward?

- Are you pigeon-toed?

- Are your ankles symmetrical?

- Are you bowlegged?

- Is your torso leaning or twisted? If you need some assistance to observe this, put your hands on your hips, then look and see if your hands are in the same place or if one is higher than the other.

- Is one of your shoulders higher than the other?

- Is your head straight or tilted?

You can also do this analysis by having someone take pictures of you from the front and from the side in your normal, everyday posture. Use the bullet points above to analyze the photos.

Freeze-Frame Exercise

For the second self-analysis, you'll take a look at your seated posture. To do this exercise, begin by sitting down, then simply freeze in place in your chair. Now look at yourself. What do you notice?

- Where are your feet?

- How are your legs positioned?

- Are your hips symmetrical with each other?

- Are your sitting bones planted in the chair equally firmly?

- Is your rib cage centered, protruding to the front or back, or tilted to one side?

- Is one of your shoulders higher than the other?

- Is your head tilted to one side, or is it forward or back from the center of your chest?

- Is there tension in your face?

- How is your breathing? Is your chest collapsed? Is your breathing deep or shallow? Is it fast or slow?

- Where do you feel the air moving in your body when you breathe?

- Are you able to take a deep breath from the position in which you are currently seated?

□ □ □

Odds are you spotted at least a few problems when you did these self-assessments—for instance, an imbalance in your shoulders when you stand or a touch of "turtle neck" when you sit. If so, don't feel bad! First of all, problems like these are epidemic in our tech-oriented era. And second, you can correct them with simple exercises. Here's how to do it.

YOUR DAILY POSTURE WORKOUT

Doing the exercises in this section will give you gorgeous posture and work out any fascial "kinks." For best results, I recommend you do all the exercises daily.

However, if you're pressed for time, know that the Wall Exercise alone will create the most lasting change. That's because this exercise doesn't just strengthen your muscles but also retrains your brain to a "new normal," so you will feel your resistance points and misalignments immediately. As you correct these, your fascia will become freer and freer.

So do the Wall Exercise daily. Then, if you have time, and you have significant posture problems or want to achieve the best possible posture, add more of the exercises in this chapter.

To get the best results from your exercise regimen, link each of the exercises with an affirmation that you repeat to yourself (see

Chapter 7). For instance, you can say one of the following silently or aloud as you exercise:

- "I feel energy coursing throughout my body."

- "I am upright, strong, and flexible."

- "I feel open, aligned, and powerful."

The Wall Exercise

This exercise will reorient your nerves and muscles to normal posture, strengthen your spinal muscles so they can help your fascia support an upright posture, train your abdominal muscles so they can work with your fascia to support correct posture, and strengthen the muscles on the back of your neck so you can hold up your head better.

To do the Wall Exercise, you need to have an empty area of wall with no pictures or knickknacks on it. Stand with your back to the wall. With your feet parallel and shoulder width apart, bring the back of your heels, your buttocks, and—if you can—your shoulders back to touch the wall. Make touching your shoulders to the wall your goal, even if you cannot do it yet.

If you can, also bring the back of your head back to touch the wall. Just be sure not to lift your nose. Your gaze should be straight on and your head level. If your head does not touch, that's okay; don't alter the angle trying to get your head to touch the wall.

If it's easy to get your head to touch the wall, do the advanced version of the Wall Exercise. If it's a struggle, do the basic version. In addition, apply a gentle, constant pressure to move your head in that direction. As you continue to do this exercise over days and weeks, eventually your head will touch. If your heels and buttocks cannot both touch the wall, step your heels an inch or two away from the wall.

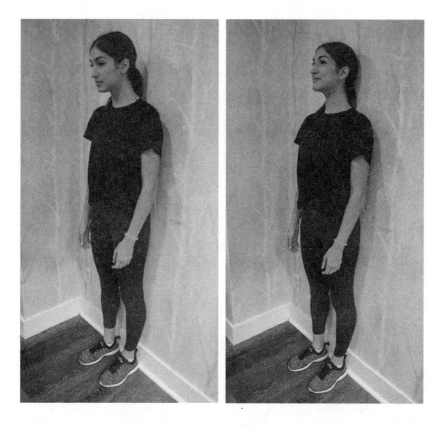

BASIC: Hold the position against the wall, then take a deep breath in and let your belly inflate like a balloon. (You can also put your hands below your belly button and use your inhale to fill your hands with your belly.) On the exhale, pull your abdominals in and toward the wall. Breathe in through your nose and out through your mouth to release tension. Remember to keep your head touching or close to the wall. Do this for 10 breaths at first. If 10 repetitions is easy for you, do 20. If 20 repetitions is easy, move to the advanced version of the exercise.

ADVANCED: Follow the instructions for the basic exercise and add pushing your head into the wall without moving your torso. This activates the muscles in the back of the neck.

The Superhero Exercise

This exercise will strengthen the muscles of your lower and upper back so they can work with your fascia to create good posture, and strengthen the muscles at the back of your neck so you can hold up your head with more ease.

Lie on your stomach on the floor. (You can also do this exercise on a bed, but the firmness of the floor is preferable unless it causes you discomfort.) Place your chin on the floor, as far forward as possible, and make a T shape with your upper arms. Bend your elbows and bring your hands in line with your ears. Your legs should be parallel, with your feet spread shoulder width apart. From this position, take in a deep breath. Then, on the exhale, lift your head, legs, and arms, squeezing your shoulder blades together.

Continue normal breathing while you are holding this position, with no extraneous movement. You should feel your back muscles working to hold you up.

To start, hold the lift for a count of 10. As you get stronger, hold it for a count of 20, then 30, and so on. The goal is to eventually build up to 60 seconds. If you feel the Superhero Exercise is strenuous, build up the time very slowly. Three to four repetitions of 60 seconds is an excellent goal.

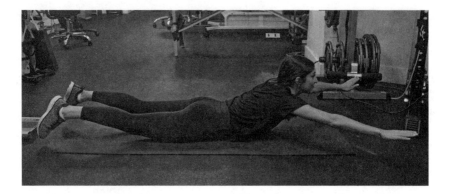

The Forearm Plank

This exercise will strengthen your core and back muscles so they can work with your fascia to promote good posture. In addition, it will strengthen your body overall so you can stand upright with ease.

Start on the floor on all fours. Lower yourself to your elbows, and rest your forearms and palms flat on the floor with your torso in a straight line. To begin, you may stay on your knees. As you get stronger, lift your knees and place your weight on the balls of your feet.

Hold the plank position for a count of 20 initially, and build to a count of 60. Do this just once per day.

TIP: Be sure to pull in your abdominal muscles, and don't collapse.

After doing the Forearm Plank, you will feel that you worked your core, abs, and back. If you feel tension in your neck or jaw, consciously relax those muscles.

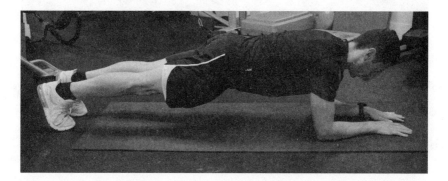

The Elbow Pushup

This exercise will open your chest, strengthen your midback, and bring your head behind your chest (which is especially useful if you need to reverse a collapsed posture).

Lie flat on your back with your legs straight. Push your elbows into the floor, bending them so your hands are pointing up toward the ceiling. Make sure your weight is evenly weighted and you are not leaning to one side or the other. From this position, take a deep breath and lift your chest to the ceiling by pressing your head and elbows into the ground. Your butt, feet, and head should stay on the floor.

BASIC: To begin, do one lift and hold it for a count of 20. Over time, build up to 60 seconds.

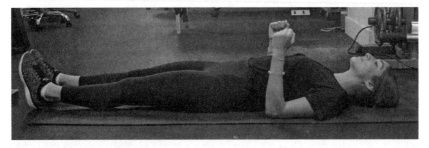

ADVANCED: Lift your arms into the air and balance on the back of your head and sacrum.

After doing Elbow Pushups, you will feel very open in your chest and feel that you have worked your upper back.

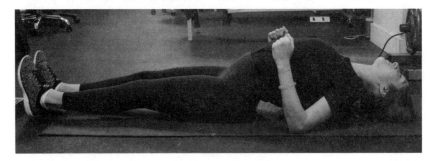

EXERCISES TO DO WITH WEIGHTS OR BANDS

If you want to take your posture to the next level, I highly recommend adding weight-bearing exercises to your daily regimen. Two of the best exercises for optimizing your posture are the Single-Arm Row and the Shoulder Opener.

When doing an exercise with weights, choose a weight that's light enough so you can do a minimum of 8 repetitions and heavy enough that you can do no more than 15. These movements are meant to be done slowly and smoothly. When using exercise bands, choose the lightest, most flexible band to begin with, and work your way up to a heavier band.

Do the following two exercises two to three times per week.

The Single-Arm Row

This exercise will strengthen the muscle that lies between your shoulder blade and spine so it can assist your fascia in creating good posture. In addition, it will help you to counter a collapsed posture.

To do this exercise, put one hand on a bench or a chair to stabilize your torso. Hold the weight in the opposite hand, which is hanging down to begin. Your spine should be long and extended. Take a deep breath. Then, on the exhale, retract your shoulder blade and bend your elbow so it points up to the ceiling. Lift the weight as high as you can, moving your hand up to your armpit. Your weighted wrist should stay straight throughout the movement.

Do 8–15 repetitions on each side. If you can get to 15 reps easily, increase the weight by a small degree.

Note: This is a back exercise, not an arm exercise. The movement should be initiated by the shoulder blade, with the arm following.

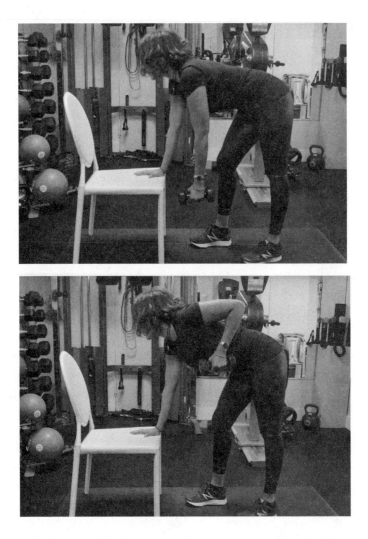

BAND EXERCISE VARIATION: Place the center of the band under your left foot and stand with feet shoulder width apart. Hold the ends of the band in your right hand, with your elbow at shoulder level and forearm parallel to the ground. Bending slightly at the waist, retract your right shoulder blade and raise your right elbow until the band is fully taut. Return to your starting position.

Do 10 to 12 repetitions, maintaining good form, and then repeat on the opposite side.

The Shoulder Opener

This exercise will counter a collapsed posture by opening your chest and shoulders and aligning your spine. It will also strengthen smaller muscles in your shoulder so they can work with your fascia to promote good posture. In addition, it will help you determine if one arm is weaker than the other and give you a means to remedy the disparity.

Stand with your feet shoulder width apart. Put a band under the inside of your left foot. Hold the other end of the band in your right hand, elbow lifted to shoulder height and forearm parallel to the floor. (Your left arm will simply rest on your side.) Now, rotate the arm holding the band so your hand is pointing straight up. Do ten repetitions on each side.

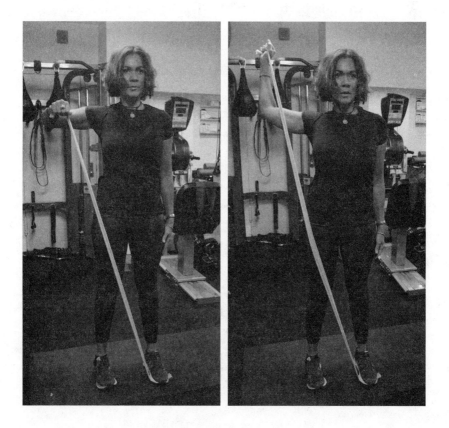

WATCH HOW YOU SIT!

At our clinic, we see hundreds of patients and clients with poor posture (and resulting fascial microtraumas and pain) caused by hours of sitting in front of a computer. If you too need to sit for most of your work day, it's important to take steps to prevent fascial damage.

One way to protect your fascia is to take frequent breaks to stretch and walk around a little. Also, stay actively aware of how you're sitting. Here are some tips:

- Starting from the bottom and working your way up, your feet and legs must be symmetrical. This might mean placing your feet flat on the floor or tucking them underneath your chair. Do not put your legs up on a bench.

- Find several good positions in which to sit. It's difficult to remain in the same position for the entire day. We aren't statues!

- Sit equally on the bones inside your buttocks, the so-called *sit bones*. When you do this, it will rock your pelvis forward and make your upright stance easy and natural to hold. If you put your pelvis at the edge of the seat, your upright sitting stance happens organically. It's easier to do this at the edge of your chair because your pelvis must come forward when you sit this way.

- Do not cross your legs. This is bad for your fascia, posture, and alignment. It can also have a negative effect on blood flow.

- You can also shift your buttocks all the way to the back of the chair and maintain an upright posture.

- Avoid sinking back into your chair. Do not roll backward and sit on your sacrum.

- Adjust your monitor so you can see it easily without holding your head in a downward position.
- To retrain your mind and body to sit upright, use affirmations (see Chapter 7) and visualize yourself sitting tall.

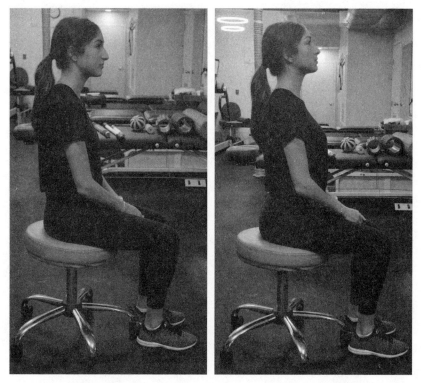

| Incorrect posture | Correct posture |

Standing and Active Desks

Also, consider using a standing desk or an active desk (used with a treadmill or stationary bike) for at least part of the day. As Dr. Cohen said earlier, "sitting is the new smoking." That's because it constricts the fascia, restricts movement, and locks our tissue into a certain position, all of which makes your fascia sick. A standing desk or active desk is an attractive alternative to hours and hours of sitting.

Here are two cautions, however:

- If you have a foot, knee, or hip misalignment or a spinal issue, standing all day can exacerbate your problem.

- Standing in poor alignment—for instance, leaning to one side—can create myofascial problems. If you use a standing desk, make sure you put equal weight on both feet. Keep your feet comfortably apart, and vary the distance between your feet occasionally.

One good tip to remember is this: Mix it up! For instance, alternate between a regular desk and a standing desk. If you have co-workers, think about getting one standing desk and taking turns with it. Remember—your fascia loves variety in movement.

CHAPTER 6

MELT YOUR TRIGGER POINTS WITH ROLLERS AND OTHER TOOLS

Rolling is one of the simplest and most low-tech therapies we offer at our clinic. But don't let its simplicity fool you, because it's also one of the most powerful and effective tools in our fascia-healing arsenal—and it should be part of your home arsenal as well.

Rolling, also called self-myofascial release (SMR), has multiple powerful benefits: it improves your performance, increases your range of motion, and can ease chronic or exercise-related pain. In addition, it's easy to do, and you only need a few simple and inexpensive tools.

Basically, SMR consists of slowly putting pressure on an area of your body with a roller, stick, ball, or other device in order to release your fascia. Alternately, you can do "static" rolling, using a ball or firm cushion to apply constant pressure to a tight area.

THE SCIENCE BEHIND ROLLING

The scientific research on foam rolling and related techniques is just beginning to emerge, but many of the early reports are highly consistent with the results we see in our clinic every day. Here's a sampling of the findings:

- One group of researchers looked at the effects of a combined program of rolling (using a baseball) and exercise on patients with myofascial pain dysfunction syndrome, a condition characterized by chronic skeletal muscle pain. Compared to a control group receiving traditional therapies, the patients in the rolling-and-exercise group experienced significant improvements in pain during daily activities.[1]

- In another study, researchers compared the effects of either static stretching alone or static stretching plus foam rolling on hip-flexion range of motion. (A control group did not do either activity.) At the end of six sessions, the group that added foam rolling to their stretching had much bigger improvements in their hip-flexion range of motion than the stretching-only group.[2]

- Examining the effects of rolling on muscle activity (remember that the muscles and the fascia are intricately interwoven), researchers asked people to either rest or do foam rolling on three consecutive days. The researchers found that foam rolling enhanced muscular activity, allowing participants to produce a given amount of force with less effort.[3]

- In a study assessing delayed-onset muscle soreness after exercise, researchers found that a 20-minute session of foam rolling on a high-density roller immediately after exercise, then 24 and 48 hours afterward, significantly reduced muscle tenderness and improved performance. "More specifically," the researchers said, "foam rolling resulted in increased pressure-pain threshold score [meaning that participants experienced less pain], sprint speed, power, and dynamic strength-endurance at various time points after exercise compared with the control condition." They concluded, "Our results provide strong evidence that foam rolling can reduce DOMS [delayed-onset muscle soreness] and the associated decrements in performance."[4]

- Researchers investigating the effects of foam rolling on the cardiovascular system concluded that it improves arterial function.[5]

- A study involving 50 participants with myofascial trigger points in the lateral gastrocnemius (calf) muscle found that static foam rolling led to relief of pain and sensitivity.[6]

THE BENEFITS OF ROLLING

While researchers are still identifying the effects of foam rolling and other SMR techniques, trainers and therapists know from experience that SMR works. That's why everyone from NFL players to Olympic athletes does it, and it's why we teach people to do foam rolling and other SMR therapies at our clinic. Here are some of the benefits our patients report:

- Less chronic pain
- Less pain after exercise
- More energy
- Better flexibility
- Greater range of motion
- Reduced stress
- Improved circulation

With results like these, it's not surprising that a survey of physical therapists, athletic trainers, and fitness professionals found that more than 80 percent of them now use foam rollers in their practice.[7]

A Word about Cellulite

Lately, there's been some talk about how foam rolling can get rid of cellulite, that dimply "cottage cheese" that forms on the thighs and butt. I haven't seen any scientific evidence that this is true, and other experts are skeptical as well.

As Sue Hitzmann, founder of the MELT Method, says: "I don't think you can 'get rid of cellulite,' just like you can't get 'rid of' your femur. The landscape of our superficial fascia has a texture to it. Can you reduce the appearance of cellulite? Sure. But it takes more than fascia therapy. It's related to hormones, estrogen, activity, nutrition, and, yes, the health of your fascia. I don't like modalities that tell people to mutilate and bruise their body to stop seeing cellulite. It simply causes unnecessary inflammation and can damage the skin overall. I think we need to embrace our form and our cellulite and love our bodies as they are."

It is true, however, that rolling will temporarily plump up these areas by driving water into the fascia and increasing circulation—so while it's not going to make that cellulite go away, it's going to make your skin look smoother in the short run.

CHOOSING FOAM ROLLERS OR OTHER SMR TOOLS

There are dozens of SMR tools you can choose from these days, from foam rollers to sticks to balls. Here's a sampling of the tools we use in our clinic:

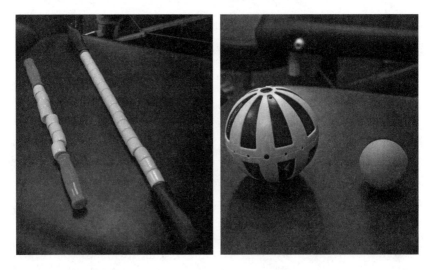

The Stick
(in two different lengths)

The Hypersphere vibrating ball
and a lacrosse ball

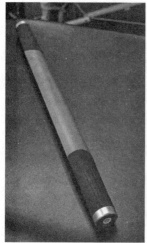

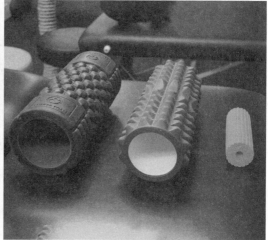

The Blackroll Releazer vibrating fascia blade

Three different types of patterned rollers

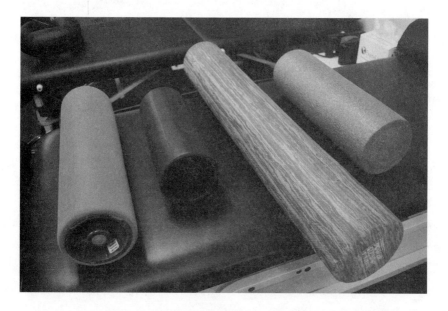

Four smooth rollers; the one on the left vibrates

The best tools for you to choose will depend on your needs. Long rollers are stable and great for areas such as your back and legs, while shorter rollers are ideal for targeting small areas like your arms. Stick rollers are excellent for working on your legs, flexible roller sticks are great for your back, and balls are an ideal tool for your buttocks, feet, and lumbar area. You can go high-tech if you want—there are rollers you can heat, rollers you can chill, and rollers that vibrate—but you can get a good basic roller or stick for ten dollars or less. You can also use a lacrosse, baseball, tennis, or golf ball.

When you use a foam roller or ball, your body's weight supplies the pressure. For instance, you can place the roller under your back, under a calf, under one hip, or under a foot. When you use a stick, you hold the stick with your hands and apply pressure where you want it.

THE GROUND RULES FOR ROLLING

Here are some guidelines for getting the most from your rolling tools:

- If you have serious chronic pain, consult with a doctor or therapist before undertaking foam rolling.

- Go slowly, so you give your fascia and muscles time to relax.

- When you're just starting out, consider using a fairly soft foam roller with no texture. As you advance, switch to a denser roller with a textured surface that creates more pressure.

- Use as much pressure as you can tolerate. Remember that your trigger points are areas of concentrated toxins, and you're pushing those toxins out. It's going to hurt a little, but it's supposed to. However, if you wind up with bruises, lighten up, because you're rolling too hard.

- Roll each area for 20 to 30 seconds at a time. When you find a particularly tender and painful spot, stay on that spot for a full minute. The prolonged pressure you apply will drive toxins out and "unstick" and loosen the fascia.

- Breathe deeply and slowly during the activity. Avoid holding your breath.

- Hydrate well both before and after rolling. Your body will need plenty of water to flush out the toxins you're releasing from the fascia.

- Foam rolling your spine is fine in general unless you've experienced a trauma there. If that's the case, be careful and get checked out by a doctor first.

- If an area is too painful to roll, work on surrounding areas.

- If you have an injury in one area and can't roll it, roll the area on the opposite side. For instance, if your right calf is injured, roll your left calf. Research shows that either rolling or stretching an area on one side can produce positive results in the other side.[8]

- Avoid foam rolling if you have osteoporosis. Also, no foam rolling near your core if you're pregnant. The joints in a pregnant woman's pelvis are relaxed in preparation for delivery, and rolling can cause problems at this time.

- Replace your roller with a new one when it starts getting worn down in spots.

POWERFUL WAYS TO ROLL OUT YOUR FASCIA

The following are my favorite ways to roll out fascial knots and restrictions. Focus on SMR techniques that address your specific areas of pain or tightness. For instance, if you have hamstring pain or tightness, roll this area daily.

If you are stiff or sore or in pain, roll the areas where you'd want someone to massage you. If the problem persists, you can roll daily. If it persists even after a few days of SMR sessions, seek professional help.

For Your Plantar Fascia (Ball)

Plantar fasciitis responds very well to rolling. For this exercise, use any small ball (a tennis ball works well). Sitting in a chair or on the floor, place the bottom of your right foot on top of the ball. Roll the sole of your foot forward and backward on the ball, gradually increasing the pressure. Repeat on the opposite side.

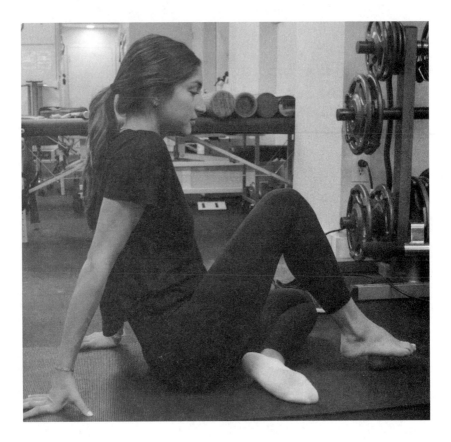

For Your Plantar Fascia (Stick Roller)

While sitting down, lay the stick on the floor, and run the sole of your right foot forward and backward over it. Repeat with your left foot.

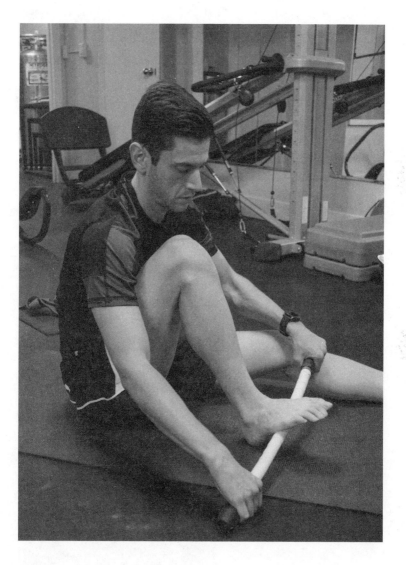

For Your Plantar Fascia (Mini Roller)

Sit in a chair with the mini-roller under your foot, leaning forward so you put pressure on the bottom of your foot. Roll the mini-roller back and forth, exerting pressure onto the roller. When you find painful areas, stay on each spot for 15 to 20 seconds. Repeat on the opposite side.

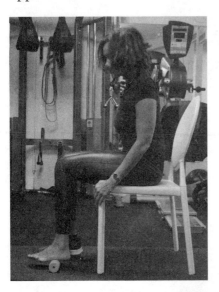

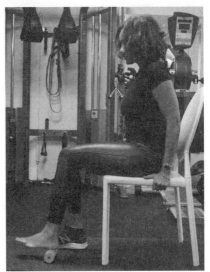

For Your Calves (Foam Roller)

Sit on the floor with your left leg extended straight in front of you and the roller under your calf. Rest your right foot flat on the floor with your knee bent. Using your hands to press your hips off the floor, roll alongside the back of your calf, from your ankle to just below your knee. Next, do this exercise with your leg rotated in at a slight angle, then rotated out at a slight angle, so you can roll along both sides of your calf. Repeat on your right calf.

For deeper pressure, do this exercise with your legs crossed.

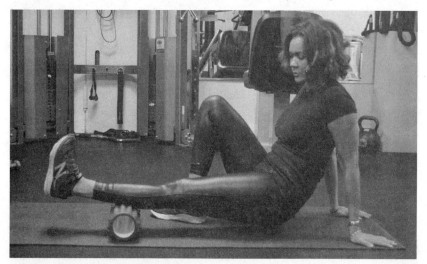

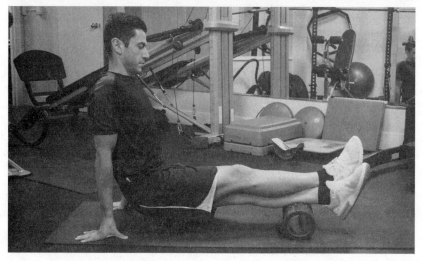

For Your Calves (Stick Roller)

Sitting on the floor with your knees bent, place the stick roller under one calf. Holding the stick with your palms facing up, roll up and down the back of your calf. Next, slightly angle the stick so you can roll the inside and outside of your calf. Repeat on the other side.

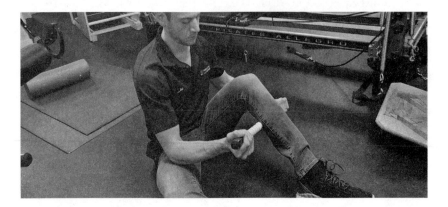

For Your Quadriceps (Foam Roller)

To work these muscles in the front of your upper legs, lie face-down on the floor with a long foam roller underneath your thighs. With your body weight on your forearms, roll yourself back and forth from the tops of your knees to your pelvis. Keep your feet off the floor the entire time.

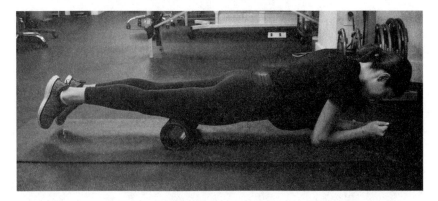

For Your Quadriceps (Stick Roller)

While sitting or standing, hold the stick across the front of your thigh and roll it up and down. Repeat with the other thigh.

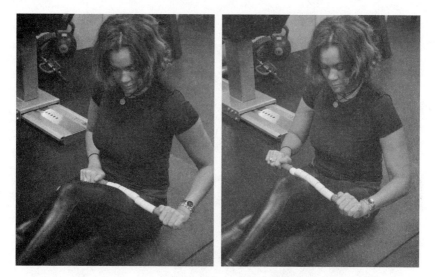

For Your Hamstrings (Foam Roller)

Sitting on the floor, place your upper thighs over the foam roller. Lifting your hips off the floor, shift your weight to your right leg. Roll over the roller, moving from below your hip to above the back of your knee and back. Repeat on the left side.

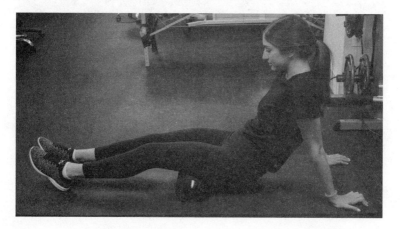

For Your Hamstrings (Stick Roller)

Sitting on the floor, hold the stick roller across the back of one thigh. Roll up and down, then repeat on the other side.

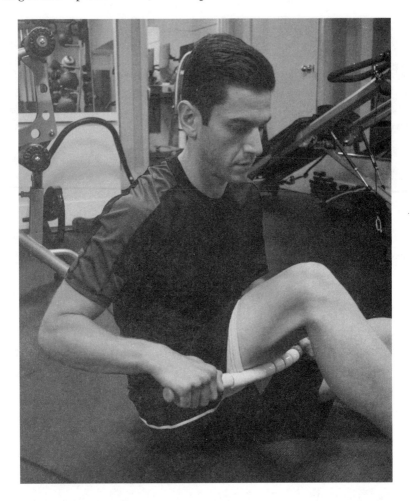

For Your Hip Flexors (Foam Roller or Ball)

Start on your hands and knees, with the foam roller or ball placed under your hips. Lower yourself until your hip flexors are lying on the roller or ball. Now lean to your right side, placing pressure on your right hip flexor. Your right leg should be straight and raised slightly off the ground, while your left leg should be bent at an angle. (Keep your left foot on the floor to provide stability.) Roll up and down for 20 seconds. Repeat on the left side.

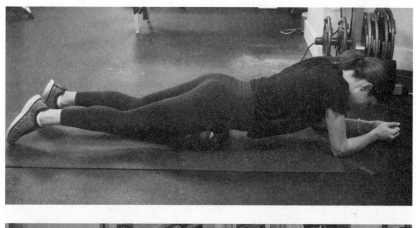

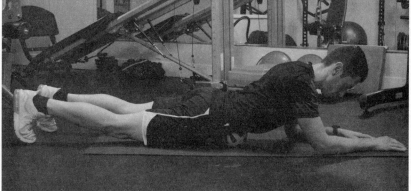

For Your Iliotibial (IT) Bands (Foam Roller)

This is a great exercise if you're a runner and have problems with your IT bands, which run along the outsides of your thighs. Lie on your right side with the foam roller under your right hip. Cross your left leg over your right leg and rest your left foot on the floor with your knee bent. Using your right forearm to move your body up and down, roll along your outer thigh from your outer hip to just above your knee. Repeat on the left side.

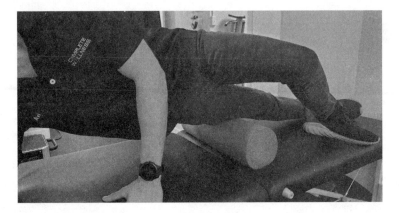

For Your Piriformis Muscles (Ball)

The fascia surrounding and infiltrating these flat, band-like muscles in your butt is a common site for restrictions and adhesions. To release them, try these exercises.

Lie on your back with your legs straight. Place a ball high on one side of your buttocks just below your waist. Lie on the ball for at least 20 seconds; longer is better. Repeat on the opposite side.

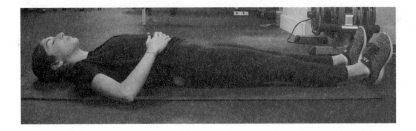

Sit with the ball under your right hip, right leg outstretched so that only the side of your right foot touches the ground. Bend your left knee, keeping your foot flat on the floor for stabilization. Lean onto your right side, and roll forward and backward along your outer hip and butt. Repeat, rotating your hips right and left as you roll. When you find a trigger point, stay on it for a full minute. Repeat on the opposite side.

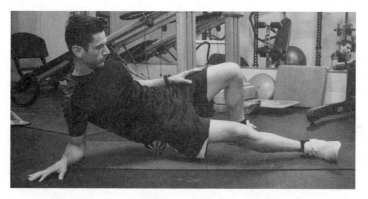

For Your Piriformis Muscles (Stick)

Kneel with your left toes and knee touching the ground, right foot flat on the ground. Roll the stick up and down your butt from your waist into the midbuttock. Switch sides.

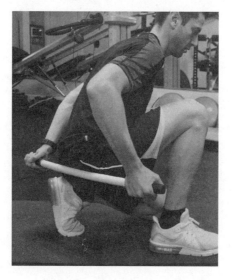

For Your Lower Back (Foam Roller)

Note: If you have lower back injuries, do not do this exercise.

Place a soft foam roller under your lower back. Roll your body up so the roller is under your hips. Use your legs to pull yourself up and down so you roll the area between your hips and upper back. Next, tilt your body to one side so you can work the sides of your back as you roll. Repeat on the opposite side. Roll for at least 30 seconds, working up to a minute each time.

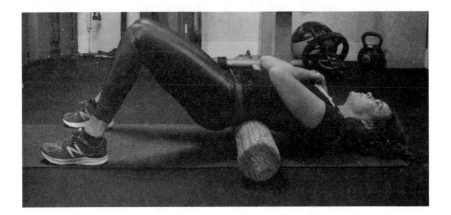

For Your Lower Back (Stick Roller)

Place the stick behind you at the small of your back and roll it slowly up and down.

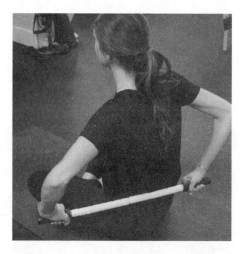

For Your Lower Back (Ball)

Lie on your back with your right leg outstretched, left leg bent, and left foot flat on the floor. Place the ball under your left hip and lie on it for 20–30 seconds.

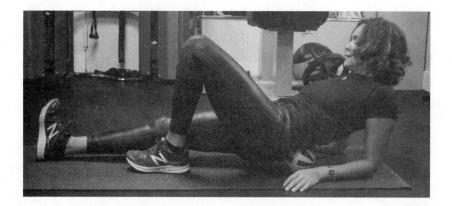

For Your Upper Back (Foam Roller)

Place the roller under your shoulders and raise your arms over your head. Your knees should be bent, and your feet should be flat on the floor. Raise your hips off the floor so they form a straight line with your upper body. Roll up and down over your shoulders and upper back.

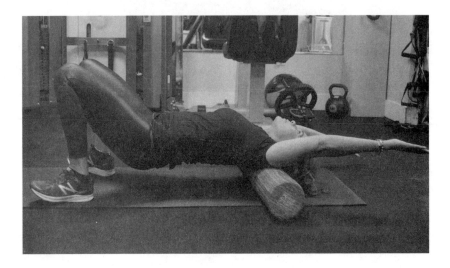

For Your Upper Back (Stick Roller)

Hold the stick behind you at a diagonal, grasping the top of the stick with your right hand and the bottom of the stick with your left hand. Roll slowly back and forth over and around your shoulderblades, in the direction of the stick. Repeat on the other side.

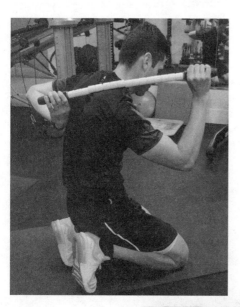

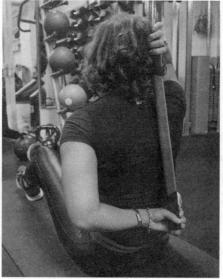

For Your Chest and Triceps (Foam Roller)

Lie on your stomach with the foam roller next to one side. Place your arm over the roller so it's resting under your armpit. Slowly roll outward and back. Repeat on the opposite side.

Next, place one arm palm up and roll along the back of the upper arm. Repeat on the opposite side.

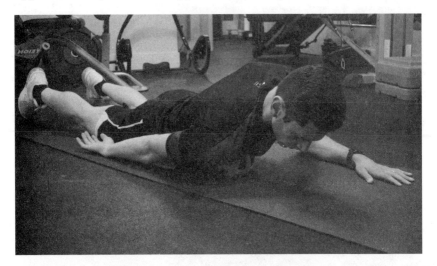

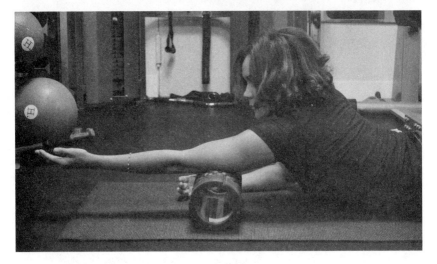

For Your Lats (Foam Roller)

Lie on your side on the floor (preferably on a yoga mat) with the foam roller under your armpit and perpendicular to your body. Extend your bottom arm straight above your head. To provide support, bend your top leg about 90 degrees. Lift your core, and roll slowly from your armpits to the bottom of your ribcage. Repeat on the opposite side.

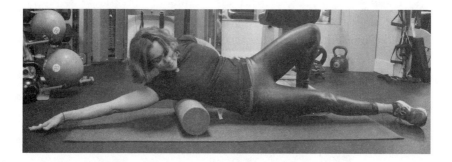

For Your Forearms (Ball)

Place a ball on a flat surface such as a table or the floor, and position your right forearm over it, palm down. Roll up and down from your wrist to your elbow, as well as in a circular motion. Then turn your arm palm up and roll the outside of your forearm. Repeat with your left forearm.

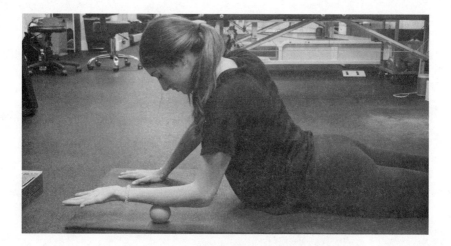

WHAT TO EXPECT WHEN YOU START ROLLING

I'm going to be honest—at first, you may actually hate your roller. That's because rolling can be a little painful initially, especially if you're stiff and sore at the outset, you overdo it, or you start with a roller that's too firm.

But stick with it, trying out different SMR tools if necessary, and you'll be very glad you did. Over time, as you free your fascia, you're going to feel less tight, less sore, and more relaxed. In addition, you'll extend your range of motion and increase your flexibility. If you're an athlete, you're also likely to improve your speed and performance—and if you spend your days at a desk, you're going to feel less tense and stressed. In short, you'll get a big payoff for a little initial pain—so if it's not love at first sight, keep rolling!

Sue Hitzmann: "MELTing" Away Fascia Problems

Sue Hitzmann is a neuromuscular therapist, exercise physiologist, and founding member of the Fascia Research Society. She is the creator of the MELT Method, a self-treatment technique for relieving chronic pain, and the *New York Times* best-selling author of *The MELT Method*. Her method focuses on balancing the nervous system and restoring the fascia's supportive qualities using gentle tools including specialized soft body rollers and small hand and foot treatment balls.

How did you get interested in fascia work?

Although fascia was discussed in all of the modalities I'd practiced in the '90s, it wasn't the primary topic discussed nor treated specifically. When I suddenly had pain out of nowhere and none of the modalities I'd learned at that time addressed the pain I had, it sent me down a path to discover what caused this sudden chronic pain in my body. The first word I typed into the Google search was *fascia*. It was 1998, and this was the start of a quest that led to my becoming a founding member of the Fascia Research Society.

As I wrote in *The MELT Method*, my understanding of fascia completely changed under the tutelage of Gil Hedley, who teaches courses on integral anatomy and dissection. Gil upended everything I thought I knew about fascia. As I searched for more research, I went down a deep rabbit hole of molecular, neurological, cellular, and noncellular science. I began to understand why our nervous system is not just some independent thing that is in charge of directing all bodily functions. Instead, our nervous system—our neurological functioning—relies on fascia, the environment it lives in, to function efficiently. Further, fascia interconnects with all our other cells, allowing them to communicate with each other so they too can function properly.

In other words, fascia has a link to neurological stability. The sudden chronic foot pain I had at the peak of my fitness career wasn't pain caused by an injury. No orthopedist knew how to fix it—because that injury wasn't in my muscles or bones. My condition also led me to understand how fascia plays a role in our sensorimotor control and our emotional stability.

What are the Four Rs of the MELT Method?

Reconnect: These are techniques we use to assess the body's current state as well as to reassess and value the changes that self-care creates. The moves we do here also help the "Autopilot"—my term for the autonomic body functions that happen without us thinking about them, such as digestion—reacquire its connection to the center of gravity. This heightens stability and efficiency in the autonomic regulators of the nervous system.

Rebalance: These are techniques that enhance the control and timing of the reflexive core and rooted core, which are mechanisms that provide whole-body balance, gut support, and spinal stability. Rebalancing techniques also recalibrate (or rebalance) the neurological regulators of stress and repair.

Rehydrate: These are techniques that restore the fluid state and supportive qualities of the connective tissue system, relieve stuck stress, and improve tensional energy. These techniques improve the environment of all the joints, muscles, organs, and bones; they also decrease inflammation in the joints and improve the fluid and nutrient absorption of every cell in the body. Compression and lengthening techniques are used to restore the elastic properties of the fascial system.

Release: These are techniques to decompress unnecessary tension and compression in the neck and low back, as well as the joints of the spine, hands, and feet. Release techniques help restore the balance between masses and spaces in the body and improve the mobility of the neck and low back space.

Tell me about the 2015 study on the MELT Method.

What's most compelling about the study overall was that the side of the thoracolumbar fascia (TLF) that was identified as more thick through ultrasound and the use of a Myoton device [which measures biomechanical properties including stiffness, elasticity, tone, and stress relaxation time] reduced in its thickness *more* than the side that was evaluated as less thick. After four weeks of MELTing, without touching the low back at all with MELT techniques, the sides evened out, which to me is why people had less low back pain. Their range of motion and stability improved; thus, better sensorimotor control and overall ease of mobility.

What kind of results have your clients experienced?

Oh gosh, there's so many. I mean, people limp in and walk out. I've had people avoid knee, hip, and shoulder surgeries, live pain-free . . . I've had people with fibromyalgia and chronic fatigue restore their overall health and well-being, getting back to an active lifestyle. Many of our instructors started with some type of chronic issue and stopped it using MELT.

How has the MELT Method been helpful for women with endometriosis?

When the pelvic floor and the uterine lining are affected by endometriosis, the pain and discomfort can be debilitating. By restoring pelvic stability and helping the tissues surrounding the viscera glide and stabilize the structures more efficiently, pain can often be reduced in this disorder.

Also, after surgeries, the fascial adhesions can be reduced through MELTing, which has been demonstrated through clients with pain from endometriosis. You can feel the difference in the tone of the tissues and sustain improvement after manual therapy using MELT.

How has the MELT Method helped people heal from emotional trauma?

Technology is allowing us to measure the bioelectrical pathophysiological regulation of the connective tissue matrix. Stimulating tissue in one area of the matrix, like a spider's web, will cause an effect through the entire web, for better and sometimes for worse. Without fascia being able to slide and glide, inflammation and irritation are inevitable during movement, and cell-to-cell communication declines.

Connective tissue is designed to stabilize joints and provide muscle support, connection, and integration so we move efficiently. But our repetitive movements and postures cause excessive tension and compression on this tissue, which causes it to lose its supportive, flexible properties. The more we repeat a motion or posture, the more the integrity of this tissue is challenged. This is a key contributor to muscle weakness, aches and pains, and a decline in performance, which can lead to an array of physical dysfunction and emotional issues.

On a larger scale, *life* just gets in the way of resilience and adaptability. Dealing with the enormous stresses of our 21st-century society creates roadblocks in our primal pathways and patterns. These roadblocks can cause our body to compensate in how it moves, accelerating body-wide issues, from joint pain to neurological or emotional disorders.

Remember, pain is your brain's way of alerting you that something is off and that you need to take action. Rather than trying to quiet down the stress regulator to restore balance, I instead worked to boost the body's repair and restore regulator. The first step was getting people back into their bodies and sensing what they were feeling.

I also realized how much our personal history can dictate how we perceive pain and react to trauma in the present moment. The energy of our emotions can influence our memories, affect our current state of feeling, and make us more worried about future events. If you take an event and connect it to an emotion, it burns in your memory, and you can recall it in an instant if another event triggers the same emotion. Often, this recall is unintentional and involuntary.

In other words, how you react to a current situation has some historical connection to how you reacted to something similar in the past. One interesting thing about the brain is that the regions where we process emotions, store past memories, and think about future intentions are also the regions where pain is processed.

Simply, MELT helps us reconnect to ourselves and focus inward, allowing our parasympathetic tone and heart rate variability to improve. Our vagal tone then regulates and allows us to manage stress with less impact to our senses.

CHAPTER 7

HEAL YOUR FASCIA BY CHANGING YOUR LIFESTYLE

Fascia is a body-wide system, so it makes perfect sense that the healthier your entire body is—and the healthier your *lifestyle* is—the freer your fascia will be. That's why this chapter is all about simple lifestyle changes that will help you heal your fascia.

If you feel a little intimidated as you read this chapter . . . don't be! You don't need to change every aspect of your lifestyle right away. Instead, make one or two changes at a time so you don't get overwhelmed. Over time, it'll all add up.

Ready to start? Here are the seven biggest steps you can take to free your fascia:

STEP 1: FIGHT BACK AGAINST AGEs

Back in Chapter 2, I talked about AGEs, the dangerous molecules that damage collagen—including the collagen in your fascia. This damage reduces the ability of your collagen fibers to slide freely, as well as dramatically accelerating aging.[1]

While your body produces AGEs naturally, you can get an overload of them from your diet. The biggest culprit here is *sugar*, so one of the most important steps you can take to heal your fascia is to cut way down on the amount of sugar you eat. In particular, wean yourself off sugary coffee drinks, sodas, and junk foods. Look at ingredient labels to find hidden sources of added sugar.

AGEs also form when you grill or broil meat at high temperatures. To counter this, you can marinate meat in an acidic marinade to significantly reduce AGE formation. Partially precooking meat at a lower heat before grilling or broiling it cuts down on AGEs as well.

Finally, reach for fresh foods whenever you can. Prepackaged foods are often high in AGEs because they're heated to very high temperatures during preparation.[2]

STEP 2: GET PLENTY OF VITAMIN C AND OTHER NUTRIENTS THAT COLLAGEN CRAVES

Fascia is largely collagen soaked in water—and as I mentioned earlier, when your body doesn't have vitamin C, it can't make collagen at all. That's why it's important to get a daily dose of vitamin C–rich foods, including berries, tomatoes, citrus fruits, kiwis, bell peppers, and dark, leafy greens. For extra insurance, consider taking a vitamin C supplement.

Also, make sure you get enough protein in your diet. The glycine, proline, hydroxyproline, and arginine in protein-rich foods are the building blocks of collagen. Foods like salmon, eggs, and bone broth are great sources of these amino acids.

In addition, eat foods like these:

- **Green, red, and orange vegetables.** These are rich in antioxidants that boost collagen production, protect collagen against damage, and help to repair collagen when it does get damaged.

- **Sulfur-containing foods.** Sulfur plays a critical role in the collagen production line. Sulfur-rich foods include onions, garlic, and brassica vegetables (bok choy, broccoli, brussels sprouts, cabbage, cauliflower, and related vegetables).

- **Hydrating foods** such as chia seeds, cucumbers, and iceberg lettuce.

- **Chlorella.** This nutrient-rich superfood binds to toxic heavy metals, helping the body to remove them.

- **Healthy fats** such as nuts, seeds, and avocados (more on this shortly).

And here's another trick: drink white tea. Research shows that it helps to counter the activity of enzymes that break down collagen.[3]

To help you start eating a fascia-friendly diet, nutritionist Liana Werner-Gray has created 20 fabulous recipes that feed your fascia the nutrients it loves. You'll find them in the Appendix in the back of this book.

The Question of Oxalates

While eating lots of fruits, vegetables, and healthy fats can protect your fascia, it's possible that some foods you think of as nutritious might harm it instead.

Health consultant Sally K. Norton, a researcher and former NIH grant recipient, has spent decades studying the potentially damaging effects of foods that contain substances called *oxalates*. If you've ever had kidney stones, oxalates (in the form of calcium oxalate) are the most likely culprit. In addition, according to Norton, oxalates may damage your bones and myofascial system.

"We see oxalate deposits in tendons," she says. "We see them causing synovitis, which is when the sheaths that cover tendons get inflamed. We see damage under the cartilage cap on bone ends—actual crystals floating around in the synovial fluid."

For many people, oxalates don't appear to be an issue. However, if you suffer from chronic neck pain, low back pain, or pain in your feet or fingers, and medical practitioners can't find a cause for it, you might want to experiment for several months by eliminating high-oxalate foods. These foods include spinach, swiss chard, beets and beet greens, nuts, seeds, and some spices such as turmeric, cinnamon, and cumin. There's a chance that it'll be life-changing.

STEP 3: HYDRATE

Remember that your fascia needs water, and plenty of it, to stay fluid. Without this water, it rapidly becomes dry, brittle, and sticky. Hydration expert Dana Cohen from Chapter 2 has plenty of tips for managing your liquid intake to keep your fascia hydrated:

- **"Front load" your water.** Start every morning with a 16-ounce glass of water. Put in a little pinch of salt for some extra minerals and electrolytes, and maybe a little lemon. (Use sea salt, Celtic salt, rock salt, or Himalayan salt rather than table salt.) You can keep a covered glass pitcher by your bedside, like Dr. Cohen does, so you can be sure to drink it first thing in the morning.

- **Drink beverages throughout the day.** To prevent dips in hydration throughout the day, drink water (still or sparkling), bone broth, and tea. And here's good news: coffee is fine too! While you may have heard that it's a diuretic, anything under four cups a day is not dehydrating.

- **Keep your electrolytes balanced.** If you drink too much water, you can affect your electrolyte levels because you're basically peeing out electrolytes and not replacing them. Dr. Cohen says that with every couple glasses of water, you should add either a commercially available electrolyte replenishment or a pinch of salt. (It has to be sea salt, Celtic salt, rock salt, or Himalayan salt as opposed to table salt. You want salt that has all the balance of the minerals in it.)

- **Have one green smoothie every day.** This will give you a big dose of hydrating gel water (more on this on page 35). In *Quench*, Dr. Cohen and Gina Bria suggest using the following ingredients to come up with your own recipe: greens, water, half an apple, a little ginger, a little lemon, and chia seeds. You'll also find a green smoothie recipe in the Appendix of this book.

- **Find out how much water is enough for you.**
  While you've probably heard that you should drink
  eight glasses of water each day, Dr. Cohen says that
  drinking half your body weight in ounces—for
  instance, drinking 70 ounces of water per day if you're
  a 140-pound woman—is a better rule of thumb.
  However, every person's body is unique. That's why
  she recommends paying attention to how you feel as
  you add water and hydrating foods to your diet. When
  your skin starts to glow, you feel more energized, your
  concentration gets better, your digestion improves,
  you sleep better, and you feel lighter and more flexible,
  you'll know that you've hit the sweet spot.

In addition to getting plenty of fluids, you can also boost your
hydration by eating the healthy fats found in natural, unprocessed
foods. These include butter, olive oil, avocado oil, coconut oil, nuts,
and the fats in oily fish, grass-fed beef and lamb, and free-range
chickens. These fats help your cells stay hydrated.

Dr. Cohen and Gina Bria explain in *Quench*, "It is oils and fats
that make cellular hydration possible. Water literally has to cross
over an oil-guarded barrier to get inside your cell. You can drink all
you want, but if water doesn't get past this membrane, hydration
isn't really happening." These membranes are constructed primarily
from fatty acids called lipids, which keep the membranes supple so
your cells can absorb water.

In particular, Cohen and Bria note, "New and important research
documents that omega-3 fatty acids play especially key roles in keeping your cell membranes supple and your cells hydrated. But that's
not all. Omega-3s can also help increase the cell membrane surface
area so that more water and nutrients can pass through."

So make sure to include healthy, hydrating fats in your diet every
day. However, avoid the hydrogenated fats used in processed foods,
which can damage and toxify your cells, leading to dehydration.
(Furthermore, processed foods "steal" water from your body because
it has to use extra water to metabolize them. Just one more reason to
stay away from them!)

STEP 4: MAKE YOUR LIFE CLEANER

Think about your fascia in the same way you'd think about your house. It's far easier to keep your house clean than it is to let it get filthy and then have to clean up the mess. Similarly, it's easier to reduce the number of toxins you put in your body (and, by extension, in your fascia) than it is to clean them out once they're there.

To reduce your body's toxic load, consider the following suggestions:

- **Purchase nontoxic and organic products whenever you can.** When you're buying household cleaners, skincare products, or cosmetics, check out the Environmental Working Group's (www.ewg.org) Guide to Healthy Cleaning and Skin Deep databases to see which products are the best.

- **Favor organic produce.** When you're buying produce, check out the EWG's Dirty Dozen list; these are the fruits and vegetables you want to buy organic whenever possible, because the nonorganic versions are heavily contaminated with pesticides. Their Clean Fifteen list, in contrast, tells you which fruits and vegetables are safe to buy in nonorganic form.

- **Invest in a good water filtration system.** Clean water is as important as clean food. Buy filtration pitchers, point-of-use filters, or—if you can afford it—a whole-house filtration system.

- **Ditch plastic.** The most important switch away from plastic that you can make is from plastic water bottles, which can leach chemicals into the water, to stainless steel or glass bottles you can fill yourself. Also consider switching from plastic food storage containers and bags to paper, glass, stainless steel, or another nontoxic material.

Dr. Sabrina Atkins: The "Magic" of Bodywork

Dr. Atkins, the founder of Orlando Sports Chiropractic, is the official chiropractic physician for the NBA's Orlando Magic and the Orlando Ballet. Her patient roster is a veritable who's who of athletes, including professional golfers, rodeo riders, power lifters, martial arts experts, and professional soccer players.

What kind of results do you see when you do bodywork with athletes?

I see crazy results all the time. For instance, people will come in after being in pain for a year and a half, and I'll treat them one time and give them some suggestions, and their pain will be 50 percent better. And after three visits, it's gone. That happens a lot because the majority of our patients are leading a healthy life. That makes all of the stuff I do easier, because a healthy body is going to respond better.

I've had situations where someone has pain in their shoulder or their knee, and I'll work on them for literally two minutes—just enough to stimulate the proprioception, increase the blood flow, activate the muscle spindles—and they have more power and less pain.

How important is lifestyle when it comes to healing? For instance, if you have two patients with the same fascia problem, how will their lifestyles affect their response to treatment?

Treatment will take much longer with a patient with unhealthy habits because I won't be able to be as aggressive. So I always assess the person and the person's situation. If I can be aggressive with my therapy, then we can work through the soreness, and they get better faster. But if someone has a little bit more going on, then I have to be a lot gentler and a lot more conservative, so it takes longer.

139

Can you share a couple of your favorite cases with us?

One patient of mine had been suffering from posterior hip pain for years, and he was at his wit's end. It had really taken a toll on his emotional health. Now, the first visit is always an assessment, so I just did a little bit of soft tissue work to see how his tissue was going to respond. By the second visit, I took him through some functional movement while on vibration and doing soft tissue work on his posterior hip. I also did a chiropractic adjustment. I tested him afterward, and it was amazing—it was miraculous. Within three visits like that, his pain was gone. And it's been gone since.

I had another guy who was a firefighter, and he had plantar fasciitis so badly that he could not walk at all—he had to hobble. It wasn't just the first 20 steps in the morning that hurt. This was a full-on "I'm in pain all day, every day" situation. The first two times I saw him, I thought he was really, really inflamed and that I needed to be gentle and flush out that inflammation, but he didn't respond. So the third time, I dug in like I was trying to dig to his bones. His problem wound up being not an inflammatory response but multiple adhesions that were stuck and tugging and creating all that pain. Once I broke up those adhesions, he was fine—and he's back to surfing and doing all the things that he loves to do.

STEP 5: MAKE SLEEP A PRIORITY

I know that getting a good night's sleep is easier said than done, especially if you're overworked or overstressed. But sleep is crucial to the health of your fascia because it gives it the downtime it needs to repair and restore itself.

In fact, the more you stress your fascia, the more sleep you need. People who are super active—athletes, dancers, and yoga instructors, for instance—require more sleep than less-active people.

What's more, if you suffer from myofascial pain, losing sleep creates a vicious cycle. That's because sleep deprivation hikes your sensitivity to pain, which in turn makes it harder to sleep. So make getting a good night's sleep a priority.

Find Out How Much Sleep Your Body Needs

Listen to your body so you'll know how much sleep it needs. Some people can get by on six or seven hours and still do well, while others may need nine or even more. To find out how many hours works best for your own body, try this strategy.

First, on a Friday night, turn off all your devices and your alarm clock, pull down the shades, and let your body wake you up when it's ready to. Then do this the next night, too. The first night, you'll be so exhausted that you'll probably oversleep. The number of hours you sleep the second night will give you a big clue about how much sleep is optimal for you.

Establishing a Bedtime Routine

To get the most benefit from your sleep, establish a bedtime routine and create a comfortable bedroom. Here are some ways to do so:

- Try to get to bed around the same time each night.

- Turn off your devices, dim the lights, and turn off the TV at least an hour before bedtime. Then read, play soft music, or take a bath. (Putting Epsom salts in your bath water will give you a dose of sleep-promoting magnesium.)

- Keep your room comfortably cool, use blackout curtains to block out light, and invest in some high-quality bedding.

- If neighborhood noise bothers you, cover it up with a white noise machine.

- Rub a little lavender oil on your bedpost.

- Journal before bedtime. Writing down your problems and thinking about ways to solve them will help you put them out of your mind at nighttime.

- Do a stretching session (see Chapter 4) an hour or so before bedtime to relax yourself and hydrate your fascia.

Optimal Sleep Positions

Also, avoid sleep positions that can cause fascial microtraumas. Here are some fascia-friendly sleeping tips:

- Avoid sleeping on your stomach, which could cause you to turn your head and neck in order to breathe. In addition, stomach sleeping causes your abdominal muscles to slacken, distorting the fascia in that area.

- If you're sleeping on your back—which is a good position—don't sleep with two pillows. This steep incline reverses the curve in your neck, leading to fascial restrictions. Instead, put one pillow under your head, and put a second pillow under your knees. This position will help take some of the strain off your back.

- If you're sleeping on your side, again stick to one pillow. Also, keep your spine straight by straightening out your head rather than tucking it forward, and bringing your knees together. Putting a pillow between your knees will also encourage good alignment.

STEP 6: DO EXERCISE—AND INCLUDE YOGA, TAI CHI, OR PILATES

Your fascia loves exercise because exercise is movement, and movement pumps the stale water out of your fascia and draws clean, nutrient-rich water in.

So any exercise, as long as you don't overdo it, is fascia-friendly. And you don't need to do intense exercise either; even small movements make a big difference. Dr. Cohen recommends incorporating micromovements throughout the day to move all of your joints—for instance, bobbing your head or doing a bicep curl without weights. However, right now I'd like to focus on three forms of exercise in particular: yoga, tai chi, and Pilates. These forms of exercise involve moving and stretching every area of your body, so they're a powerful way to refresh your fascia from head to toe. In addition, they involve *slow* movements, which are the best types of movements for pumping water in and out of the fascia. So it's no wonder that all three do wonders for your fascia, leading to reduced pain and improved balanced and flexibility, among other effects. Here's a sampling of reports from the research:

- In a study that enrolled physiotherapists with neck pain as participants, researchers found that a yoga program "led to significant improvement in the quality of health, physical capacity (strength), cervical range of motion, and pressure threshold of the trigger points [the pressure at which discomfort occurred], and decreased . . . disability and pain."[4]

- Another study found that just 12 weeks of tai chi relieved chronic fibromyalgia symptoms and improved the quality of life for people with this disorder. One researcher involved in the study commented, "We definitely saw better results than reported in trials of drug treatments for fibromyalgia. . . . One patient with previous arthritis pain kept saying, 'No pain! No pain!'"[5]

- In a study involving 228 adults with chronic low back pain, researchers divided participants into three groups. Two groups did either yoga or stretching exercises, while the third group read a self-care book describing the causes of back pain and suggesting lifestyle changes to reduce pain. The researchers reported that compared to the controls, people in both the stretching and yoga groups had significantly less pain and used less pain medication both at the end of the study and at a later follow-up.[6] A related study found that yoga was as effective as physical therapy in easing chronic low back pain.[7]

- In a meta-analysis of studies on the effects of Pilates on breast cancer, researchers found that it improved shoulder range of motion, quality of life, pain, and upper extremity function.[8]

143

- A study investigating the effects of Pilates on chronic pain in patients with a range of medical problems found that it "enabled the participants to function better and manage their condition more independently."[9]

- Researchers report that at-risk or older adults who practice tai chi can reduce their risk of falls and injury-related falls by 43 percent and 50 percent, respectively.[10]

Clearly, your fascia loves these forms of slow movement, so do it a favor and add at least one of them to your exercise routine.

Dr. Howard Sichel: Energizing the Fascia with Pilates

Dr. Howard Sichel, a chiropractor, is the founder and former owner of Power Pilates, the world's largest education company teaching classical Pilates. Named after Joseph Pilates, who invented the approach, Pilates is designed to stretch, balance, and strengthen the body. Recently, I talked with Dr. Sichel (who, incidentally, is a cousin of mine) about the powerful effects of Pilates on the fascia.

When did you first hear about Pilates?

In 1982, I was introduced to classical Pilates by a woman I'll call MP, who was a master teacher of coordinated dance. This woman was probably in her early 70s, and her posture was impeccable. Her stature was beautiful. Everything about her was incredible. However, because of her age and her complaints, I did take x-rays. To my surprise, they showed severe degenerative osteoarthritis throughout her cervical, lumbar, and thoracic spine.

In chiropractic school, we learned that you diagnose and do treatment protocol based on what your tests and x-rays show. It didn't make any sense to me that MP's movement and her posture did not mirror what the x-rays showed. We got to talking, and I said, "What do you do physically besides dance?"

She said, "Pilates." I learned that she'd been a devout student of Romana Kryzanowska's classical Pilates for years.

So I met Romana, and I started referring people to her. I immediately noticed that these people, once I initially relieved their pain, no longer needed to see me as often. They saw me for maintenance and balance work, but not for acute or chronic weaknesses.

You started doing Pilates yourself and eventually opened your own studio. As you got into Pilates, what surprised you the most about it?

It really took time for me to understand what classical Pilates was. It wasn't merely about muscle. It was about using all the apparatuses to challenge the body, to challenge the muscles and tendons, the ligaments and the fascia. Of course, no one knew about fascia back then. All I knew in my own practice was that I started working on soft tissue because I wasn't satisfied with only adjusting the bones. I realized that I had to go above and below the area of complaint and work on soft tissue to release tension. I didn't know it then, but I was working on fascia.

Can you tell me a little about Pilates?

The goal of Pilates is to improve joint function, range of motion, posture, and spinal health. Originally, it was developed just as mat exercises and exercises using a person's own body. Then Joe Pilates realized that in order to make it easier for people to do, as well as challenge them at the same time, you needed equipment. Now Pilates uses apparatuses to challenge the body, to challenge the muscles and tendons, the ligaments and the fascia, through the use of springs and the movement of different pieces of equipment.

In Pilates, no exercise is held. You move right through a whole sequence. So the fascia gets released and energized throughout the whole body. There isn't one exercise; it's a whole series of 55 minutes of exercises that really energizes the person.

> When people come out, they feel different. The correc-
> tions are dramatic, and they happen in a very short period of
> time.
>
> **How does Pilates specifically affect the fascia?**
>
> When you have poor posture, energy doesn't flow. As a
> result, the fascia isn't as vibrant as it needs to be. When you
> improve posture, all of a sudden the energy within the fascia
> can really start to "vibrate." The circulation and energy within
> the fascia flow more freely when it isn't restricted or con-
> stricted as a result of poor posture or poor joint function.
>
> A human body is all about energy—and the only way to
> battle the effects of aging and chronic weaknesses is through
> movement that releases and energizes the fascia.

STEP 7: TACKLE YOUR STRESS

When you stress out, your fascia stresses out right along with you. Stress causes your fascia to contract, leading to tightness, knots, and poor hydration—so one of the best things you can do for your fascia is to dial down your stress.

Many people feel tempted to skip this step, thinking it's not as important as nutrition and sleep, for example. Dr. Brett Ander-son, however, looks at it as mind hygiene—cleaning our minds of all the junk that's out there. "If collective thought is fascia, and we want fascia to be healthy, then we should be doing things that promote positive thoughts," he says.

Luckily, there are simple techniques you can use to cut your stress down to size. These strategies are quick and easy, but they're also very powerful. Recently, researchers tested the effects of a combination of stress-fighting techniques on some of the most stressed-out people on the planet: spouses caring for husbands or wives with dementia. In the study, they asked the caregivers to do these eight things every day:

- Identify one positive event that occurred each day.

- Tell someone, either in person or via social media, about the positive event, allowing the caregivers to enjoy the event all over again.

- Start a daily gratitude journal, listing large or small things for which they were grateful. (This is one of my personal favorites.)

- Identify a personal strength and reflect on how they had used this strength recently.

- Set a daily goal—one that was simple and doable—and track their progress.

- Practice "positive reappraisal" by identifying an unpleasant daily event or activity and reframing it in a more positive light. One caregiver, for instance, reframed her stressful outings with her husband as a positive thing by realizing that it was good that they could still take outings together.

- Perform a small act of kindness for someone else each day.

- Practice mindfulness by paying attention to the present moment.

The study found that after just five weeks of using these strategies, participants' anxiety scores and depression scores dropped by 14 percent and 16 percent, respectively, compared to a control group. They were also healthier and felt more positive about life and about their caregiving role.[11]

Affirmations to Relieve Stress

Another great stress-reducing strategy we teach our patients is to use *affirmations*. Put simply, an affirmation is a way to focus your conscious and unconscious mind on positive thoughts and banish negative and stressful ones. Louise Hay, one of the most important pioneers in self-healing, said, "An affirmation opens the door. It's a beginning point on the path to change. In essence, you're saying to your subconscious mind: *'I am taking responsibility. I am aware that there is something I can do to change.'"*[12]

Remember that *everything your body does is controlled by your brain.* Negative self-talk leads you to expect failure, which ramps up your stress. Positive self-talk does the exact opposite: it helps you feel in control, reducing your stress.

Thanks to modern imaging techniques, we can actually see the effects of affirmations happening inside the brain. A few years ago, researchers asked a group of adults to undergo functional magnetic resonance imaging while thinking positive affirmations about the future. Compared to a control group who focused on thoughts not related to affirmation, the self-affirmation group showed greater activation of key reward pathways in the brain. These brain changes translated into real-world changes, correlating with greater success by participants in improving their lifestyles later on.[13]

We like to think of affirmations as "exercise for your brain"— and as with physical exercise, you'll get the most benefit if you make affirmations a part of your daily routine. For instance, tell yourself one of the following:

- "I am in control of my life and will make good decisions."
- "I am taking action to make my body and my fascia healthy."
- "I am changing my diet in ways that are making my fascia freer."

You can integrate affirmations into the routines of your daily life—for instance, when you're washing dishes, brushing your teeth, or getting ready for work. If you're waiting in line at the grocery store or you're stuck in traffic and you want to fill your time by doing something useful, repeat your affirmations. Any time you have a negative thought, use an affirmation to turn it into a more positive thought.

Mindful Meditation to Relieve Stress

Modern science is catching up to what hundreds of years of tradition have shown: meditation offers a cascade of physical and mental benefits, including stress relief. Here are some simple steps to start meditating today.

- Find a quiet place where you won't be interrupted. Leave your phone and any other devices in another room.

- Sit quietly in a comfortable position on a chair, cushion, or mat, with your eyes either open or shut. Breathe slowly and deeply, focusing on the sensation of the air entering and leaving your body.

- As thoughts enter your mind, don't fight them, even if they're negative. Instead, examine each thought, and then gently let it float away. Then return your focus to your breathing. You may find it helpful to utter a phrase or word with each exhalation.

- At the end of your meditation period, pause for a minute or two to pay attention to your environment and your own body—for instance, what you hear, what you see, how warm or cool your body is, and what emotions you're feeling. Then think about what you want to do with the rest of your day.

When you first start meditating, your mind may race, and you may find it hard to simply sit still. However, keep practicing, and it'll become second nature.

If you feel like you're too busy to set aside time to meditate, do what's called "moving meditation." When you're walking the dog, doing housework, or mowing the lawn, pay attention to your breathing, your surroundings, and your own physical and emotional feelings. Be "in the moment" rather than focusing on getting the chore done. When you do this, you'll refresh your mind and spirit—and at the same time, you'll be able to check off another item on your to-do list.

To Lower Your Stress, Be a Jerk!

Here's one more tip for reducing your stress: be a jerk. No, I don't mean kick the cat or yell at your kids. When I say "be a jerk," I mean stop pushing yourself all the time. Every once in a while, say, "I'm not going to do anything productive for the next two hours. I'm just going to chill." Then lie in bed, go window-shopping, binge-watch a show on Netflix, or organize your sock drawer. The lazier you are, the better.

Many of us have the pedal to the metal all the time—I know I'm frequently guilty of this myself—but you can't keep driving the car when it's out of gas. So don't keep pushing yourself to the limit in an effort to be perfect. Aim for 80 percent, and you won't drive yourself (and your fascia) crazy.

Most people wait for a vacation or the weekend to be a jerk, but by that time, you may be running close to empty. Having a little regular weekly "jerk time" in your life can be a game changer.

TAKE THE FIRST STEP

Each positive lifestyle change you make will lead to a happier, healthier fascia. So right now, pick your first goal and commit to following through on it. Once that lifestyle change becomes habit, pick your next goal. In time, you'll be eating better, hydrating more optimally, reducing your exposure to toxins, getting better sleep, exercising more, and stressing out less—and all of that will do your fascia a world of good.

CHAPTER 8

Tackle Serious Fascia Problems with the Aid of Professionals

So far, I've talked about ways to free your fascia on your own, from stretching to foam rolling to lifestyle changes. However, if you have moderate or severe fascia problems, now is not the time to rely solely on do-it-yourself therapies (although these can still help). In this case, it's crucial to team up with professionals who can identify and treat the root causes of your issues.

What's more, getting help quickly matters. That's because, left untreated, serious myofascial problems typically don't get better over time—they get worse.

Remember that restrictions in one part of your body start to affect other areas, causing a cascading effect. For instance, if you have plantar fasciitis in one foot and let it go untreated, you'll begin to walk with an uneven gait in an attempt to protect that foot. As a result, you can develop trigger points in your legs, your back, and even your neck.

So don't procrastinate and hope that "maybe it will go away." The sooner you get help, the smaller your problems will be and the easier it will be to resolve them.

COLLABORATIVE CARE

When it comes to professional help, there's no one-size-fits-all solution. At our clinic, for instance, we may design completely different programs for a professional athlete with a knee injury and a middle-aged office worker with the same problem. Like these patients, you need treatment designed for your unique issues, abilities, goals, and lifestyle.

This is why I recommend going to an integrative medicine center if you can. At a center like this, professionals won't just give you prescriptions or cookie-cutter advice. Instead, they will work hard to uncover the roots of your problems and design a program that addresses them with natural, drug-free, noninvasive or minimally invasive techniques. In addition, they will approach your problems from as many different angles as possible. One angle is good, but not as good as two or three or four.

Integrative wellness centers like ours typically have a large staff, including professions such as the following:

- Integrative medicine doctors: If you visit a center like ours, this will typically be the first person you'll see. This doctor will take a thorough history, do an evaluation, and order tests. Based on all of this, a personalized plan can then be created for you.

  Note: Doctors may have an M.D. (doctor of medicine) or D.O. (doctor of osteopathy). A doctor with a D.O. is called an osteopath or osteopathic physician. Either degree allows a doctor to practice medicine in the United States. Generally, a D.O. undergoes the same training as an M.D., along with studies in osteopathic manipulation.

- Physiatrists/rehab doctors: This is a medical doctor specializing in helping patients with injuries or disabilities. Physiatrists are nicknamed "quality of life" doctors because they focus not just on a specific injury but on every aspect of a patient's life— emotional, social, and occupational. At centers like ours, the physiatrist develops a treatment plan and also collaborates with a patient's other doctors to coordinate care.

- Chiropractors

- Physical therapists

- Acupuncturists

- Massage therapists

- Personal trainers with special training in stretching and/or fascia work

- Instructors in yoga, Pilates, tai chi, and other forms of fascia-friendly exercise

- Nutritionists and/or health and nutrition coaches

- Fascia specialists (including experts in Rolfing, Feldenkrais, and the Alexander technique)

Your plan is likely to involve several additional specialists, and each of these people will have different roles to play in healing your fascia. Practitioners in different fields that affect the myofascia often debate their version of the chicken-and-egg question: What came first, vertebrae out of alignment or tight muscles? Is bad alignment causing the muscles to tighten? Are tight muscles pulling on the vertebrae? Is nerve impingement causing constriction of the muscles? The answer is: Yes—all of these are happening. And does it matter? No. That's because the complete solution will address both the myofascial tightness and the misaligned vertebrae.

This chapter offers a look at some of the most common myofascial treatments that integrative medicine centers offer.

Christina Howe: Rolfing and the Fascia

Christina Howe is the executive director of the Dr. Ida Rolf Institute, which teaches the myofascial techniques developed by Dr. Rolf in the early 1900s.

Tell me a little about Rolfing.

The bottom line is that Dr. Ida Rolf recognized that fascia played a bigger role in integrative health than we realized. She also realized that gravity is a unilateral force on the body, and that this force—sometimes compounded by injuries or even by embryological issues—can result in people having imbalances in their bodies, such as pelvic imbalances or a forward head thrust or a ribcage that's out of alignment.

You know that we as human beings are designed to have our bodies be stacked on top of ourselves in a line. But because of forces of gravity, injury, or even emotional impacts on our lives, we can get out of alignment. So Dr. Rolf started looking at holistic ways to bring the body into better balance with gravity, to free up energy and make the body more at ease.

Dr. Rolf developed a series of 10 sessions, called the Ten-Series, to accomplish this. The initial sessions focus on the lower body, and on stabilizing us and connecting us with the earth. Then we move into sessions where we look at the center of the body, from the pelvis up into the chest and neck. Next, we work on the upper body, from the shoulders to the head. And then the last three sessions are integrated. Rolfing really involves working from the ground up, connecting the feet to the head, and looking at how that all of those segments work in unison together.

You say that a large part of the work of a Rolfing practitioner involves educating people. Why is that?

We don't Rolf people to stand in the corner; we Rolf people so they can move through life. So teaching people about movement and how to reinhabit their bodies with new patterns is a powerful part of this work. I think it sets us apart from many other types of touch therapies. All of them are good, but I think Dr. Rolf recognized that really educating people to *inhabit* those new patterns, being very intentional and developmental about it, is as big a part of the work as the structural work.

What types of problems can you address through Rolfing?

Everything from cerebral palsy to post-traumatic stress. There's work on multiple sclerosis and arthritis as well. Rolfing seems to cause global improvements. There's something about the *whole-ism*—working on the fascia and aligning the body and gravity—that eases the body and seems to trigger a healing mechanism.

Ida Rolf wrote that while Rolfing isn't primarily a psychotherapeutic approach, it can provide emotional as well as physical release. Has this been your experience?

It does seem to be the case that when some people are Rolfed, there is a dramatic emotional release. That can happen with massage as well. It can even happen with dance. Whether the body holds trauma at a cellular level or at a fascial level or at the muscular level, there does appear to be a memory system there that can be released through touch.

CHIROPRACTIC ADJUSTMENT

Chiropractic is rooted in an understanding of health as emanating from the spine and its associated muscles and fascia. This is a longstanding principle; in ancient Greece, Hippocrates, the father of western medicine, said to "look to the spine for the cause of all disease."

On many levels, chiropractic care comes down to *posture*, meaning that people's alignment is optimized when their posture is at its best. Ultimately, the goal of chiropractic care is to improve a person's posture and alignment.

When a person has bad posture, it puts tremendous stress and strain on the soft tissue. For example, when a person has "turtle neck," the muscles and fascia that connect the base of the skull to the shoulders and mid back are put under enormous stress (see my comments about "text neck" on page 31). This causes microtrauma. When we correct alignment and posture, we restore the myofascial tissue to a healthier state.

Chiropractors adjust all the bones and joints of the body, but our primary focus is the spine. The bones and joints of the spine and the myofascial tissue are intimately connected, so any kind of adjustment to the spine is going to positively affect the surrounding myofascial tissue. It's probably impossible to adjust vertebrae without affecting myofascial tissue.

Research shows that chiropractic treatment is highly effective. For example, one group of researchers comparing the results of chiropractic treatment of lower back pain to the results of back pain treatment provided by general practitioners reported, "Patients with chronic low-back pain treated by chiropractors showed greater improvement and satisfaction at one month than patients treated by family physicians. . . . A higher proportion of chiropractic patients (56 percent vs. 13 percent) reported that their low-back pain was better or much better, whereas nearly one-third of medical patients reported their low-back pain was worse or much worse."[1]

Chiropractic treatment often eliminates the need for surgery—especially back surgery, which can be dangerous and often fails to reduce pain. A 2015 study of people with back injuries found that "reduced odds of surgery were observed for . . . those whose first provider was a chiropractor. 42.7% of workers who first saw a surgeon had surgery, in contrast to only 1.5% of those who saw a chiropractor."[2]

Patients' use of addictive opioid drugs can also be dramatically reduced with the use of chiropractic. In one recent study, researchers examined insurance claims data from the state of New Hampshire (which has the second-highest age-adjusted rate of drug overdose deaths in the United States). They found that among people with non-cancer-related low back pain, the likelihood of filling a prescription for an opioid analgesic was 55 percent lower for those using chiropractic services than for those not receiving chiropractic treatment.[3]

In addition to improving posture and reducing pain, chiropractic adjustments can increase your flexibility, improve your balance, and help your entire body function more efficiently, all at a fraction of the cost of medications or surgeries. It's no wonder that about 33 million Americans visit a chiropractor's office in a single year.[4] They're part of what's dubbed the "chiropractic first" movement: people who want to try safe, effective, noninvasive, and inexpensive treatments before (or instead of) resorting to risky operations or potentially addictive drugs.

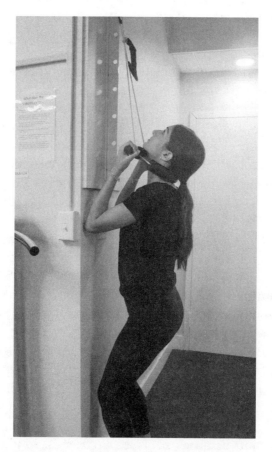

Pettibon Cervical Stretching: This chiropractic stretch is very effective for relieving neck and jaw pains.

The Patient Who Got "Ripped"

Like many people, I never really enjoyed stretching. I knew it was important, but I didn't do it because it didn't feel good.

Then, years ago, I discovered a procedure called *active isolated stretching*. I first learned about it from *Whartons' Stretch Book*, which my wife—an exercise physiologist and trainer—shared with me. In this approach, you hold a stretch for only a few seconds, rather than the minute or so of static stretching.

I discovered that this dynamic type of stretching, which works on the superficial and deep fascia planes, felt better and was easier to do than static stretching. Even better, I loved the results. I became a client of the Whartons and eventually wound up working as a clinician at their center, where I incorporated isolated active stretching into my chiropractic practice.

In addition to learning isolated active stretching from the Whartons (see page 6), I studied it under Aaron Mattes, the expert who created the procedure. And one piece of wisdom he shared with me came in handy just a little while later, saving me from a moment of pure panic.

At one point when he was demonstrating a stretch, Mattes said to me, "Sometimes you'll do this, and you'll hear a sound like paper tearing." I was like, "Sure. Whatever." Frankly, I thought it sounded pretty far-fetched.

The very first patient I saw after that was a man named Ken. He was a good candidate for active isolated stretching because he had neck pain, was very round-shouldered, and jutted his head forward. However, during the third or fourth repetition of stretching Ken's right trapezoid muscle I heard what sounded like a phone book ripping. Ken exclaimed, "What was that?"

I instantly thought, *Did I just break something?* Fortunately, I remembered what Aaron had told me. I reassured Ken that everything was fine, and we both relaxed. And then he said, "*Wow*—that feels so much better."

I've heard that sound many times since then. Now, however, it doesn't scare me, because I know it's a *good* sign. So if it happens to you, don't panic . . . it just means your fascia is getting freer.

CUPPING

When Michael Phelps made a big splash at the 2016 Olympics, so did a myofascial intervention he used called *cupping*. Instantly, the technique caught on with everyone from professional and Olympic athletes to Hollywood celebrities. But while cupping is a new trend, it's also a very old practice, dating back to 1550 BCE in Egypt and 20 CE in China.

In cupping, a practitioner seals a cup to the skin of the target area for around 2 to 15 minutes, using a vacuum pump or heating the cup to create a vacuum inside the cup that gently lifts the skin away from the underlying tissue. Dr. David Hashemipour, who does cupping at our clinic, explains that this procedure separates the adhesions between the fascia and the muscle. "In addition," he says, "we increase perfusion. After cupping, lots of blood rushes to that area, and it becomes red. That hyper-perfusion is a reaction that helps in detaching adhesions and is also anti-inflammatory—like cleaning the area."

Dr. Hashemipour was part of the team treating athletes at the 2016 Olympics, and one of his favorite memories is treating a swimmer with a restriction in the trapezius area the day before the swimmer's competition. The swimmer was concerned because he knew the restriction would hurt his performance on the big day. After cupping and acupuncture (see next section), Dr. Hashemipour says, "he said, 'Oh—it's completely gone!' And he was super happy."

In addition to its anti-inflammatory effects and its effect on perfusion, researchers have other theories about why cupping works. One is that it breaks collagen cross-linkages. Another is that it activates mechanoreceptors in the fascia.[5]

Whatever the reason, research shows that cupping has significant effects. For example:

- A 2019 study involving 21 healthy young participants found that cupping improved the range of motion in participants' hips and knees.[6]

- In another study, patients with low back pain reported significant improvements in pain and range of motion after undergoing cupping. The researchers commented, "Chinese cupping may be a low-risk, therapeutic treatment for the prompt reduction of symptoms associated with subacute and chronic low back pain."[7]

- Scientists studying the effects of cupping on carpal tunnel syndrome compared one group of people who received only physiotherapy to a group that underwent physiotherapy and cupping. Participants in the cupping-plus-physiotherapy group showed a significant improvement in symptoms compared to the physiotherapy-only group.[8]

- Researchers reviewing 18 different studies on the use of cupping for neck pain say the studies showed that cupping significantly reduces pain, enhances function, and can improve quality of life.[9]

Done correctly, Dr. Hashemipour says, cupping doesn't hurt. It may leave a mark for 24 hours, but the mark should not last beyond that.

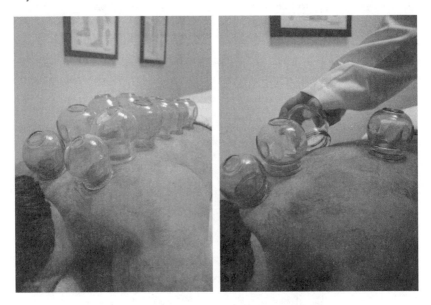

Cupping equipment and marks left by cupping

ACUPUNCTURE

In addition to doing cupping at our clinic, Dr. Hashemipour performs acupuncture—another modern technique that has ancient roots.

In fact, Dr. Hashemipour notes, early practitioners of Chinese medicine were among the world's first fascia therapists. "When we insert the needles through the skin, it is very important where we stop," he says. "In Chinese medicine, this is the root of acupuncture. It's not just putting in the needle; you need to know how far to put it in. Two thousand years ago, they didn't know about this term, *fascia*. But in the books, they said, 'Under the skin and before the muscle.' And the fascia is exactly there."

Thanks to research by Helene Langevin and colleagues, we now know the remarkable effect that acupuncture has on the fascia. Several years ago, the researchers looked at the microscopic effects of rotating an acupuncture needle in a piece of rat abdominal wall. In a feature in *The Scientist*, Langevin commented, "What we saw under the microscope was quite striking: when acupuncture needles were rotated, the loose connective tissue under the skin became mechanically attached to the needle. Even a small amount of rotation caused the connective tissue to wrap around the needle, like spaghetti winding around a fork. This winding caused the surrounding connective tissue to become stretched as it was pulled by the needle's motion. Using ultrasound, we confirmed that the same phenomenon occurs in live tissue.[10]

Additional research is revealing that the stimulation resulting from acupuncture starts a chemical cascade including a decrease of inflammatory cytokines, an increase of T lymphocytes, and increases in adenosine, neuropeptides, opioid peptides, peptide hormones, and stem cells.[11] So it's no surprise that acupuncture has powerful and wide-ranging effects, from easing back pain to alleviating headaches.[12]

MASSAGE THERAPY

Myofascial therapies frequently combine the best of traditional and modern medicine, and massage is a perfect example.

Textbooks from China written nearly 5,000 years ago describe massage techniques. Ancient writings and paintings from Egypt, Japan, Greece, and India also show practitioners doing massages.

Today, using modern tools, we're learning more and more about the science behind the powerful effects of massage. For instance, we now know that massage alters EEG patterns, the activity of the vagus nerve, and levels of cortisol.[13] Functional magnetic resonance imaging shows that massage can also cause changes in brain regions, including the amygdala, hypothalamus, and anterior cingulate cortex—regions involved in stress and emotional regulation.[14]

The benefits of massage are extensively documented in hundreds of studies. Here are just some of the findings about its effects:

- A study involving patients with chronic low back pain found that compared to usual care, massage resulted in more effective pain relief, fewer days in bed and days off work, and less use of nonsteroidal anti-inflammatory medications. The researchers added, "Most notably, 36%–39% of participants receiving massage, versus only 4% receiving Usual Care, claimed their back pain was much better or gone."[15]

- In another study, 15 women with cancer were asked about the effects of aromatherapy massage. The researchers reported, "The perceived benefits of aromatherapy massage included physical and psychological dimensions: overall comfort, relaxation, reduced pain, muscular tension, lymphoedema and numbness, improved sleep, energy level, appetite and mood."[16]

- A separate group of researchers assigned 46 adults with hand pain to receive massage therapy or standard treatment. The researchers reported, "Over the four-week period the massage group had a greater decrease in pain and a greater increase in grip strength as well as lower scores on anxiety, depressed mood and sleep disturbance scales."[17]

- Investigating the effects of massage on exercise-related injury, researchers administered either massage therapy or no therapy to 11 young men with acute quadriceps damage resulting from strenuous exercise. They reported that "when administered to skeletal muscle that has been acutely damaged through exercise, massage therapy appears to be clinically beneficial by reducing inflammation and promoting mitochondrial biogenesis."[18]

- Patients who suffer serious burns often have painful, itchy scars. A study of 146 burn patients found that adding massage therapy to their rehabilitation programs significantly decreased scar thickness, pain, itching, and redness.[19]

- Around one third of people with multiple sclerosis use massage therapy in addition to other medical treatments, and recent research showed that massage can effectively reduce pain and fatigue in people with MS.[20]

Massage therapists use a variety of techniques, including gliding strokes, kneading, friction, compression, percussion, and vibration, to free myofascial tissue. Depending on your needs, there are dozens of different types of massage to choose from—everything from a gentle and relaxing Swedish massage to a deep tissue massage targeting adhesions and scar tissue. There are even massages specifically designed for athletes, pregnant women, or seniors.

At a clinic like ours, your massage therapist will assess your medical needs to determine the right kind of massage for you. If you don't have access to an integrated wellness center and you're new to massage, you may want to start with a Swedish massage.

When you get a massage, ask your therapist to point out trigger points you can massage yourself, and have the therapist show you how to do this. Adding "do-it-yourself" massaging to professional treatments will give you even more benefits.

PS: One of the most common questions people ask about medical massage is, "Do you need to take off all your clothes?" The answer is that you can, but you don't need to. So if you're modest, there's no need to avoid the massage table.

THERAPY TAPE

Watch any major sporting event, and you'll spot athletes wearing colorful tape on their arms, legs, backs, or feet. The tape isn't there for decoration; it's there to improve the athletes' performance and reduce pain from injuries.

Therapy tape recoils when it's placed on the skin, pulling the skin away from the fascial tissue. Steven Capobianco, co-founder of RockTape, compares this to lifting the skin like a handle. Musculoskeletal ultrasounds reveal that therapy tape lifts the skin one to three millimeters, creating significantly more space for tissues to glide.

Professionals use taping to treat myriad problems, including the following:

- Knee injuries
- Shin splints
- Hamstring injuries
- Plantar fasciitis
- Tennis elbow
- Back pain
- Rotator cuff injuries
- Wrist injuries

In addition to relieving pain, therapy taping can provide support and stability, reduce the risk of injury, soften scar tissue, improve circulation, and promote drainage of the lymph system. Professionals also use it to improve posture by "reeducating" the body to stand and sit straight, rather than slumping.

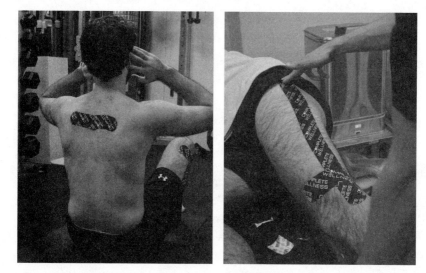

Taping the back to promote
upright posture

Taping the leg to reduce IT
band pain

The original therapy tape, Kinesio Tape, was invented in 1977 by Dr. Kenzo Kase, a Japanese chiropractor, but therapists now have multiple types of tape to choose from. Initially, doctors were skeptical about the benefits of taping. Now, however, studies are revealing its benefits:

- In a study involving 65 pregnant women with low back pain, the women received acetaminophen only or a combination of acetaminophen and taping. The researchers concluded that "the Kinesio taping group was significantly superior to the control group in all outcome measures."[21]

- Another study, this one involving 43 participants who underwent either active or placebo taping for low back pain, found that fascial taping "reduced worst pain in patients with non-acute non-specific low back pain during the treatment phase."[22]

- A study involving women found that taping on the anterior surface of the thigh increased quadriceps strength during isokinetic exercise.[23]

- Investigating the effects of hand taping in women, researchers found that it augmented hand grip strength, an effect that lasted for 48 hours after application.[24]

- A study comparing two treatments for plantar fasciitis—shockwave therapy and Kinesio taping—found that both improved pain, function, and quality of life.[25]

- Researchers exploring the effects of Kinesio taping on lymphedema following mastectomy found that it reduced swelling and pain, improved hand grip strength, and enhanced quality of life for participants.[26]

Another interesting study involved 32 surgeons. Surgeons spend hours in very awkward positions, keep their heads held forward and down for long stretches, and work in a tense, high-stress job—a "perfect storm" of issues that lead to myofascial distress.

In this study, the doctors performed surgery without taping on some days and with taping on other days. The surgeons reported that they felt much less pain in their necks and low backs on the days they wore the tape, and tests showed that they had a greater range of motion. The researchers commented that even after the study ended, the surgeons kept coming to them for taping before performing long surgeries.[27]

Unlike tape that immobilizes part of the body, therapy tape leaves the body free to move. The tape comes in different tensions, and a therapist will select a tape with the correct tension to address your specific myofascial issues. It's waterproof, so you can wear it when you're swimming or showering, and it lasts several days, extending the benefits of a therapy session.

In addition to its immediate benefits, therapy taping can relieve pain even after the taping is stopped. Recently, Capobianco told me, "The goal is not to become dependent on the tape, but instead to condition the brain and the nervous system to accept that you can move without pain."

TRIGGER POINT INJECTIONS

Trigger point injections are injections directed into tense muscles called *taut bands*. These bands contain "knotted" areas of fibers that make the muscle extremely tight and lock up toxins inside it.

When a needle goes through the fascia and into a taut band in a muscle, the muscle will twitch. This twitch happens when the tense fibers release, unlocking the toxins and allowing the tight muscle to stretch. Because muscle and fascia are intimately connected, this release occurs in the fascia as well.

Trigger point injections can contain lidocaine or another local anesthetic to help relax the muscle and fascia further. However, the twitch and release occur even in "dry needling," which doesn't involve an anesthetic.

Doctors or physical therapists can use trigger point injections anywhere in the body where there is fascia or muscle, as long as there isn't any bone in the way. The cervical thoracic region (the neck and upper back) tends to be the most common location because people spend a great deal of time in a forward-flexed head position that strains the muscles and fascia in this area.

Trigger point injections aren't just a temporary fix; they are also powerful preventive medicine. At our clinic, we use them in combination with physical therapy to help patients strengthen muscles and stretch tight fascial bands to create a relaxed, balanced body alignment. This can prevent future muscle spasms and keep trigger points from developing.

Because multiple studies and reviews show that trigger point injections are safe and effective, physicians are increasingly recommending them to patients.[28] Doctors writing in the *Journal of the American Board of Family Medicine*, for instance, have encouraged family practitioners to consider this intervention, noting, "Dry needling is a treatment modality that is minimally invasive, cheap, easy to learn with appropriate training, and carries a low risk."[29]

Trigger Point Therapy and Acupuncture: What's the Difference?

Both acupuncture and trigger point therapy (called dry needling when no anesthetic is used) involve needles. However, there are big differences between the two.

Acupuncture is an ancient practice based on traditional Chinese medicine. Trigger point therapy, developed in the West, became popular just a few decades ago. Acupuncture addresses problems ranging from pain to stress to insomnia, while trigger point therapy specifically treats myofascial pain and tightness.

In acupuncture, which is designed to balance the flow of energy throughout the body, a practitioner inserts needles into *meridian lines*—energy pathways in the body—leaving the needles in for up to 15 minutes. A practitioner doing trigger point injections, in contrast, leaves a needle in just long enough to achieve the twitch that shows that the muscle has released.

Interestingly, while the two approaches are very different, research done by Peter Dorsher at the Mayo Clinic shows that acupuncture points and trigger points are anatomically and clinically similar.

In one study, Dorsher found that at least 92 percent of common trigger points correspond anatomically with acupuncture points, and more than 95 percent correspond clinically. "That means," he said, "that the classical acupoint was in the same body region as the trigger point, was used for the same type of pain problem, and the trigger point referred pain pattern followed the meridian pathway of that acupoint described by the Chinese more than 2,000 years before."[30]

VIBRATION

One popular myofascial technique is whole-body vibration, which involves sitting, standing, lying, or doing exercises on a vibrating platform. The vibration puts all of your myofascial system in motion, giving you a head-to-toe workout. It's great for balance and circulation, and it's popular with athletes because it can improve balance and agility and help to prevent or treat muscle soreness after workouts.[31] (As a bonus, vibration helps with building bone, which is why astronauts use vibrating platforms to counteract the bone-thinning effects of being in space.) Therapists might also use vibrating foam rollers or a vibration gun to target trigger points. Here is a vibrating platform we use at our clinic.

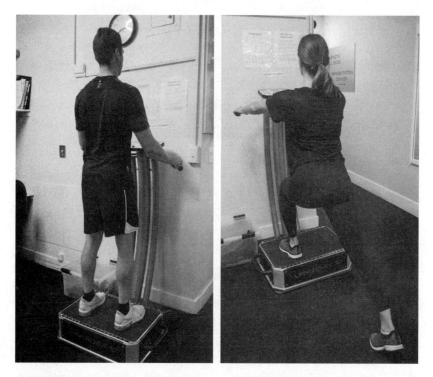

Standing on a vibrating platform

A lunge stretch on a vibrating platform

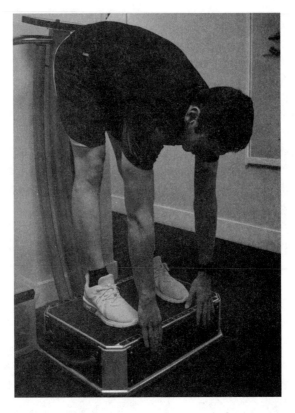

A forward stretch on a vibrating platform

ORTHOTICS

Orthotics are custom-molded insoles placed inside a person's shoes. These insoles, which correct abnormal arches in the feet by placing them in a neutral position, often ease fascia problems throughout the body—not just in the feet.

Physiatrist Shilo Kramer, D.O., who frequently prescribes orthotics at our center, explains, "When a patient has a very flat arch or a very high arch, the increased forces through the bottom of the feet will actually have repercussions not just on the plantar fascia but also on the legs, knees, thighs, hips, and back. When you place the feet in their normal position, you're taking pressure off the fascia and off specific muscles. So orthotics aren't just about additional cushioning for people who walk or stand a lot. There's actually a corrective component to them."

In addition to using orthotics to correct abnormal arches, we use them to correct an imbalance in leg length. Here's a sampling of the orthotics we prescribe at our clinic:

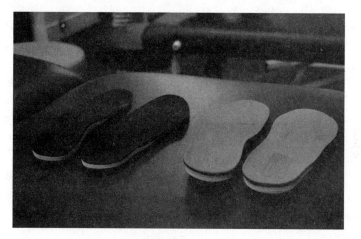

Two different types of orthotics

LIFESTYLE APPROACHES

Remember Dr. Dana Cohen's patient, Betty, back in Chapter 2? To cope with the pain caused by fibromyalgia, Betty started to drink heavily. With the help of Dr. Cohen, Betty's pain went away, and so did her drinking problem.

Conversely, lifestyle problems—for instance, obesity or a lack of exercise—can cause someone to develop fascia problems. For instance, DJ, the weekend warrior I talked about in Chapter 1, developed serious pain as a result of sitting too much during the week and then overexercising on the weekends.

This is another of those chicken-and-egg problems. Whether a myofascial problem leads to lifestyle issues or lifestyle issues lead to a myofascial problem, the smart approach is to address both. This is why the professionals at an integrated wellness center won't just address your physical problems. In addition, they'll help you identify any lifestyle issues that contributed to these problems.

What's more, you'll get advice that's designed specifically for you. For instance, at our clinic, nutritionist Liana Werner-Gray customizes a nutrition plan for each patient she sees. She says, "In my ten-plus years of coaching thus far, I've found that no nutrition plan is exactly the same. None! It's all individualized based on the health history of the patient, their health goals, blood type, their cravings, addictions if any, brain activity, budget, sleep patterns, exercise status, the season, and where they live. All of this is factored in. That's why their nutrition plans are successful: because the plans are exactly tailored to them, and if anything needs to be changed along the way, I change it."

In addition to helping patients reduce strain on their fascia by losing weight, nutritionists can help them plan a diet that's rich in fascia-friendly foods. "A person with a healthier diet will have healthier fascia," Werner-Gray says. "A nutrient-rich diet provides adequate vitamins and minerals so the fascia can do its job." In particular, she says, a nutritionist can show you how to add anti-inflammatory foods to your diet and reduce your intake of pro-inflammatory foods, "because inflammation is one of the most common fascia problems caused by diet."

The good news, Werner-Gray says, is that changing your diet can be easier than you think—even if you're a junk-food enthusiast. "I ask patients about their favorite foods and talk about how they can make these foods healthier and more nourishing for the body and fascia," she says. "This works especially well for people who love fast food, fried food, crackers, and chocolate, because there are so many delicious recipes and products that fulfill these cravings without damaging the body."

One key to healing the fascia with diet, Werner-Gray says, is to be patient and give your body time. For instance, she talks about a recent patient I'll call Mia. "I gave Mia a customized nutrition plan and assured her that she would achieve her weight loss goals if she followed it," Werner-Gray says. "She struggled at first, but I kept encouraging her to implement one small thing at a time, reminding her that it takes time to transform the body, including the fascia. I told her if she kept going, she would see results. After six months, she became discouraged, as she only lost a few pounds, which is quite common because the body is initially busy absorbing so many nutrients and rebuilding the fascia. Then, finally, she started dropping the pounds, and she lost 50 pounds in the next six months and has been able to keep it off."

In addition to offering nutritional services, most integrative wellness centers offer the services of personal trainers and instructors in yoga, Pilates, and other forms of exercise. These professionals can design a program that any patient—even someone with fibromyalgia, severe arthritis, or other serious physical problems—can follow with ease. This allows us to give patients the *successful movement experiences* that Dr. Brent Anderson notes are crucial to improved well-being (see page 67).

A lifestyle coach can also be a key part of your team. Along with helping you address areas of your life where you're experiencing difficulties, this professional can teach you simple but powerful tricks—for instance, affirmations and mindful meditation—that can dramatically reduce your stress level.

Jeff Migdow, M.D.: Yoga and Fascia

Jeff Migdow, M.D., has taught yoga since 1969 in places as varied as the U.S., India, Japan, Canada, Brazil, Colombia, and Peru. He directed and taught Kripalu Yoga Teacher Training from 1990 to 1997 and developed Prana Yoga Teacher Training, which he directed at the Open Center in NYC from 1997 to 2013 and at the Princeton Center for Yoga and Health from 2013 to the present.

Dr. Migdow has been practicing holistic medicine since 1980. His practice in Lenox, Massachusetts, offers homeopathy, herbal treatment, lifestyle counseling, and Reiki healing and attunements. He has written and taught widely about yoga and holistic health and medicine, including the Time-Life book *Breathe In, Breathe Out* with Dr. James E Loehr and is the co-author with Sierra Bender of *Goddess to the Core*.

How does yoga affect the fascia?

If you have good alignment when you go into the postures and you're breathing fully and deeply while you're in the pose, and you hold the posture, your fascia will stretch out. When you release, the fascia is much more expanded than it was before you started the pose.

So it's about movement, holding, breathing.

Yes. For instance, many of the teachers doing an aerobic style of yoga don't focus on breathing at all. So I might be holding and holding for a long time, but if I'm not breathing, then the structural system is actually getting more tense. And when I release, I really won't get much of an expansion in the fascia, because of the tension created.

On the other hand, if I'm doing yoga where I'm breathing slowly and deeply, but I'm not holding, I'll get relaxation in the whole system, but I won't get nearly as much stretch, because I'm moving from one position to the next. For instance, if I'm stretching the fascia in my arm, but I'm not really holding it but instead moving to another part of the body, then the fascia in my arm will contract back. If I'm holding it for a period of time, then it can stay more stretched out.

All forms of yoga are good. But in terms of fascia, it's my experience that if you're not doing the breathing, the tension that you build up is just going to snap it back. And if you're not doing the holding, it's a little like blowing up a balloon a little bit and letting the air out over and over again. It's not really going to stretch at all. But if you blow the balloon up fully and then hold that air in for a while, then when you release the air, the balloon's going to be more stretched than when you started.

So if someone is very tight and really wants to increase their range of motion, you might suggest Hatha yoga for the long holds?

Yes. Today, most styles of yoga are more exercise-ish. You're not really able to relax into a pose and hold it. The relaxing and holding not only helps stretch the fascia but also relaxes the fight-or-flight response in the nervous system, which allows the whole structural system to relax to a deeper level.

Any tips for getting the most fascial benefit from a yoga workout?

If you don't do warm-ups before you do your postures, you'll just get a quick stretch, and it'll pop back. So it's always good to do at least 10 or 15 minutes of warm-ups first.

Also, it's important not to have sugar or coffee right before or after a workout, because that stimulates the flight-or-fight response, and the muscles and fascia will tighten up. Some people go to class, then they'll go to Starbucks after that. And they'll have a nice yoga experience. But their structure really won't be much more flexible than it was before they started.

You've seen a lot of patients over a lot of years. What's the most surprising response that you've seen in your practice?

I guess the most unexpected response involved a woman from Pennsylvania who was in her 70s. She had severe arthritis in her joints. Because of that, the muscles became tight around her joints to protect them.

Her fascia was so constricted that she could barely walk, not just because of the pain but also because she was extremely stiff. She had to walk up a single step to get into my office, and I had to help her because she couldn't even do that by herself.

We worked with some homeopathic remedies to relax her system, but mainly we focused on simple warm-up stretches and gentle yoga. It was barely yoga, but it was breathing and holding, and she really was persistent. She said to me, "You know, if I can't move because my body hurts so much, that's one thing. But if I can't move because it's gotten so *tight* because my body hurts, I just can't accept that."

I saw her every month for about six months, and by then she could go up and down stairs and move much more easily. About three months after our last session, she sent me a postcard from one of the highest suspension bridges in the country. She had traveled there with a friend, and she was able to climb up the hill to get to the top of that bridge. On the postcard, she wrote, "Thanks a lot for helping me to experience this magnificent view!"

In her case, I just was hoping she would be able to walk across the street and go up and down a few stairs. But she was very persistent.

So I guess the message is that there is real hope even for people with chronic conditions.

For sure. Of course, one key for her was that I'm a physician too. If we'd just practiced yoga, she could have reached a certain point, but she still would have had pain that would have kept her to a certain level. Because we could also work with her diet and homeopathy, we were able to greatly diminish her pain. On the other hand, the stretching alone created more space around the joints that also diminished the pain. She received a double benefit.

Any other stories from your practice?

Some of the people who go through the Prana Yoga Teacher Training have severe arthritis or have deep injuries or autoimmune diseases. Usually by the third or fourth weekend, their body is shifting. The first weekend, many of the students aren't very flexible in their yoga practice. By the third or fourth weekend, I feel like I'm teaching a really solid group of students in the classes. They open up structurally, and even the way they walk is different. It's really wonderful to see.

GETTING STARTED

Knowing where to start when you're seeking professional help for fascial problems isn't always easy. That's why I recommend going to an integrated wellness center, where the staff can develop a coordinated care plan for you. If you don't live in an area large enough to have such a center, I recommend starting with an osteopath, a physiatrist, or a massage therapist.

Also, seek out health-care professionals who don't just offer temporary symptom relief but also ask, "Why is this happening—what is the cause?" and "How can we correct the cause?" The best way to get real help for myofascial problems is to find a practitioner who's willing to search for the roots of problems.

The other day, for instance, I asked a patient about her bunion, and she said, "I'm having surgery for it in November." I asked, "Wouldn't it be interesting to know where the bunion came from—if you have some kind of pelvic or spinal misalignment putting pressure on the joint?" And she said, "Oh, yes, I just found out that I have scoliosis." I explained that while bunion surgery would get rid of the problem temporarily, it would be wise to address the cause so the bunion didn't come back!

It's true that in rare cases, easing symptoms temporarily with drugs or surgery is the best we can do. But most of the time, it's possible to *fix* a problem. That fix might not always be 100 percent, but it's not zero percent either—and the more you reduce a problem, the less it will impact your life. So look for a practitioner who wants to know not just *what* your problem is but also *why* you have it.

Also, don't fall into the trap of being a passive patient. Ask questions, and make sure you understand the answers. When you understand the causes of your problems and the goals and approaches of a practitioner, you will be an active partner in your care, and that leads to the best results.

Most important of all, don't wait any longer to begin healing your fascia. Get started today, either on your own or with a professional team on your side. Now that you know about your body's largest and most intriguing organ, you're ready to treat it with the respect it deserves.

AFTERWORD

The Fascia Revolution

No matter where you are right now—whether you have serious fascia problems, you want to nip minor problems in the bud, or you're an athlete seeking to take your skills to a higher level—taking charge of the health of your fascia can be life-changing. As the evidence in this book clearly shows, healing your fascia can reduce your pain, increase your flexibility, improve your balance, enhance your mood, and optimize your posture and performance. You can address everything from crippling joint problems to agonizing back pain to sports injuries to fibromyalgia—and you can do it all in a safe and oftentimes noninvasive way.

What's more, you'll be at the forefront of a revolution in medicine. Over the next 20 years, I believe that we will see astonishing developments in the field of fascia: new ways of quantifying the fascia, new ways of treating fascia-based problems, and even new ways of preventing disease through optimizing fascial function. More and more people will make stretching, rolling, hydrating, and other fascia-healing techniques part of their health regimens. Increasing numbers of people will say no to dangerous drug treatments for pain and instead embrace acupuncture, chiropractic, massage, and other forms of bodywork. And you will be a part of this movement, because you are a member of the first generation to fully understand the significance of this mysterious and magical organ.

Welcome to the fascia revolution!

APPENDIX

Fascia-Friendly Recipes

Feeding your fascia can be delicious! I asked Liana Werner-Gray, a nutritionist at our clinic and the author of *Cancer-Free with Food*, *10-Minute Recipes*, and *The Earth Diet*, to share some of her favorite fascia-healing foods. Here they are:

CLASSIC GREEN SMOOTHIE

Total time: 5 minutes • Makes 2 servings

1½ cups nut milk or filtered water (your choice)

2 cups kale

1 frozen banana

1½ cups blueberries

1 cup spinach

1 serving of chlorella or chlorophyll supplement

Put all the ingredients in a blender and mix until it reaches a smooth consistency.

□ □ □

GREEN LEMONADE

Total time: 10 minutes • Makes 1 serving

2 apples

1 large cucumber

1 large celery stalk

1 (roughly) thumb-size piece of ginger

½ large lemon, peeled

Put all the ingredients in a juicer. Juice and drink.

Serve over ice cubes, if desired.

□ □ □

BERRY GREEN JUICE

Total time: 10 minutes • Makes 1 serving

1 cup blueberries

1 cup strawberries

1 small cucumber

1 large celery stalk

1 handful of kale

1 handful of fresh cilantro

¼ lemon, peeled

Put all the ingredients in a juicer. Juice and drink.

TIP: Juice a 1-inch piece of turmeric with the other ingredients to boost the juice's anti-inflammatory properties.

□ □ □

CHOCOLATE CAULIFLOWER SMOOTHIE

Total time: 10 minutes • Makes 1 serving

1 tablespoon cacao powder

1½ cups almond milk

3 seedless dates or 1 tablespoon honey

1 cup frozen cauliflower

½ large frozen banana

Pinch of sea salt

Dash of vanilla extract

Put all the ingredients in a blender and mix until it reaches a smooth consistency.

TIPS:

- Try adding a scoop of protein powder.
- To cut down the sugar intake, substitute an equal amount of frozen cauliflower for the frozen banana. (I prefer to use half cauliflower and half banana.)

□ □ □

ENERGY TEA

Total time: 10 minutes • Makes 2 servings

4 cups filtered water

1 teaspoon dried green tea leaves

1 small handful of fresh
mint or 1 teaspoon dried mint

1 teaspoon ginseng root or
powder

Boil all the ingredients in a saucepan for 5 minutes.

Strain the liquid as you pour it into teacups. Drink warm.

□ □ □

MEDITERRANEAN OMELET

Total time: 10 minutes • Makes 4 servings

2 tablespoons extra-virgin
olive oil

8 eggs

¼ cup olives, sliced

1 cup spinach

1 small tomato, sliced

1 small handful of fresh parsley

1 teaspoon minced garlic

Handful of organic cheese
or nutritional yeast

Pinch of sea salt

Heat the coconut oil in a large pan.

Whisk the eggs in a bowl, then pour them into the pan.

As the egg mixture starts to firm up, top it with the olives, spinach, tomato, parsley, garlic, cheese (or nutritional yeast), and sea salt.

When the bottom of the omelet is cooked and firm, use a spatula to fold it in half. Let cook until interior is at desired consistency.

□ □ □

ULTIMATE SUPERFOOD SMOOTHIE

Total time: 10 minutes • Makes 2 servings

2 cups almond milk or tigernut milk

1½ teaspoons pure vanilla extract

½ cup blueberries

½ cup kale

½ cup broccoli sprouts

1 tablespoon goji berries

3 seedless dates

3 figs

2 cups ice

½ teaspoon maca powder

½ teaspoon mangosteen powder

1 teaspoon pomegranate powder

½ teaspoon bee pollen

½ teaspoon spirulina

¼ teaspoon cacao powder

1 teaspoon coconut oil

1 teaspoon hemp seeds

1 teaspoon chia seeds

1 teaspoon flaxseeds

¼ teaspoon turmeric powder

Put all the ingredients in a blender and mix until it reaches a smooth consistency.

□ □ □

PROTEIN BALLS

Total time: 10 minutes • Makes 15 balls

7 tablespoons almond butter

½ cup almond meal

¼ cup collagen

5 tablespoons raw honey or maple syrup

3 tablespoons hemp seeds, plus extra for topping

3 tablespoons pumpkin seeds

Mix all the ingredients until they are moist enough to stick together. If the mixture feels too dry to mold, add more water.

Form the mixture into balls, then roll in hemp seeds.

□ □ □

BLUEBERRY CHIA SEED PUDDING

Total time: 10 minutes • Makes 2 servings

1 cup fresh blueberries, plus extra for optional garnish

2 cups almond milk

½ teaspoon vanilla extract

2 tablespoons honey or maple syrup

¼ teaspoon sea salt

½ cup chia seeds

Blend all the ingredients together except the chia seeds and garnish.

Add the chia seeds and then set in fridge for 9 minutes so the pudding can gelatinize. Check the consistency, and if it is not at desired doneness, let it set for an additional 20 minutes.

Serve with fresh blueberries, if desired.

□ □ □

ENERGIZING FIVE-INGREDIENT GREEN SALAD

Total time: 10 minutes • Makes 1 serving

1 avocado

1 cup fresh parsley leaves

1 cup fresh cilantro leaves

1 cup broccoli sprouts

1 lemon

Chop the avocado into cubes. Place the cubed avocado, parsley, sprouts, and cilantro in a bowl. Squeeze the lemon over the salad, and mix gently.

TIPS:

- Add sea salt and pepper to taste.
- Include the stems from the parsley and cilantro for added nutrients.

□ □ □

SUPERFOOD KALE SALAD

Total time: 10 minutes • Makes 3 servings

1 bunch of kale, center ribs and stems removed (save the stems and ribs for juicing or eating later)

1 avocado

1 tablespoon apple cider vinegar

1½ tablespoons flaxseed oil

¾ teaspoon sea salt

4 tablespoons nutritional yeast

4 tablespoons sunflower seeds

3 tablespoons pumpkin seeds

½ teaspoon garlic powder

Tear the kale leaves into small pieces and place in a large bowl. Massage the avocado into the pieces of kale with your fingers, covering the kale with avocado.

Add the remaining ingredients to the bowl and stir, or continue to massage the mixture with your fingers, until everything is well combined.

□ □ □

CHICKPEA CUCUMBER CUMIN SALAD

Total time: 5 minutes • Makes 4 servings

For the salad:

1 cup chopped kale

¼ cup chopped spinach

¼ cup chopped broccoli sprouts

1 large cucumber, cubed

One 14-ounce can organic BPA-free chickpeas

For the seasoning:

1 teaspoon cumin

¼ teaspoon sea salt

Cracked black pepper, to taste

Smidgen of turmeric powder

1 tablespoon black seeds

For the dressing:

Juice of 1 lemon

2 tablespoons olive oil

Divide the kale, spinach, broccoli sprouts, and cucumber among 4 salad bowls. Drain the chickpeas and add those on top of the greens.

Mix the seasonings in a bowl and sprinkle evenly over each salad.

Mix the lemon juice and olive oil for the dressing. Pour over the salads and serve.

□ □ □

ORANGE ARUGULA AVOCADO SESAME SEED SALAD

Total time: 10 minutes • Makes 2 servings

For the salad:

1 orange, peeled and sliced

2 cups arugula, torn into pieces

1 slice of purple onion, in wafts

1 avocado, peeled and sliced

¾ cup snap peas

1 tablespoon roasted sesame seeds

½ teaspoon black seeds

Garnish with fresh parsley, cilantro, and ½ cup broccoli sprouts

For the dressing:

1 teaspoon sesame seed oil

2 teaspoons olive oil

Dash of sea salt and pepper

Juice of ½ lemon

1 tablespoon orange juice

Layer the salads on 2 plates, starting with the orange slices. Then add the arugula, followed by the onion, the avocado, and the snap peas.

Make the dressing by whisking the ingredients together in a bowl and pour over each salad.

Finish by sprinkling the salads with the seeds, fresh herbs, and broccoli sprouts.

□ □ □

GRATED BEET AND CARROT SALAD WITH SUNFLOWER DRESSING

Total time: 10 minutes • Makes 2 servings

For the salad:

4 carrots

1 small beet

1 tablespoon fresh basil

For the dressing:

3 tablespoons apple cider vinegar

1 tablespoon Sunbutter (sunflower seed butter)

Peel and grate the carrots and beet by hand or with a food processor. Slice the basil and add to a bowl along with the vegetables.

Mix the apple cider vinegar and Sunbutter in a separate bowl and whisk until thick and creamy. (You can also use the food processor for this step.) Pour over the salad and toss until well coated.

□ □ □

KIDNEY BEAN SOUP WITH WATERCRESS AND KALE

Total time: 15 minutes • Makes 4 servings

1½ tablespoons coconut oil

1 brown onion, chopped

1 teaspoon garlic powder

3 cups filtered water

1 cup vegetable broth

Two 15-ounce cans organic kidney beans, rinsed and drained

2 cups kale, diced

2 cups watercress, diced

¼ teaspoon cumin

Black pepper to taste

Handful of broccoli sprouts

Heat the oil in a large saucepan over medium-high heat. Add the onion and garlic powder and cook for 1½ minutes.

Add the remaining ingredients and cook for another 12 minutes. Season to taste with cracked black pepper.

Serve and top with broccoli sprouts.

□ □ □

TURMERIC CUMIN QUINOA BOWL

Total time: 25 minutes • Makes 3 servings

1 tablespoon cumin

½ teaspoon turmeric powder

1 teaspoon sea salt

1 teaspoon extra-virgin coconut oil, extra-virgin olive oil, or sesame oil

1 teaspoon black pepper

Dash cayenne pepper, if you like a little kick

One avocado, chopped into cubes

One large cucumber, chopped into cubes

½ cup cilantro

¼ cup broccoli sprouts

Strawberries, for garnish (optional)

½ lemon

Add the quinoa and 2½ cups of filtered water to a pot. Bring to a boil over high heat.

Reduce the heat to low, cover, and simmer for 15 minutes. The quinoa will absorb the water during the process.

Add the remaining ingredients and continue to cook, stirring occasionally, for another 3 minutes, or until the quinoa is soft and all the flavors are well combined. Add quinoa to bowls.

Place the avocado and cucumber alongside the quinoa in a bowl. Sprinkle with cilantro and broccoli sprouts, as well as strawberries if desired.

Squeeze lemon over each bowl, and it's ready to enjoy!

□ □ □

BAKED WALNUT-CRUSTED SALMON

Total time: 35 minutes • Makes 4 servings

1 cup walnuts, blended to a meal

1 teaspoon sage

½ teaspoon sea salt

1 teaspoon thyme

1 egg

1½ pounds of skinless salmon, cut into 4 pieces

Handful broccoli sprouts

Preheat the oven to 380°F.

Prepare a baking sheet with parchment paper or a thin coating of coconut oil.

Mix the walnut meal, sage, sea salt, and thyme in a bowl. Beat the egg in a separate bowl and dip each salmon fillet into the egg. Press each fillet into the walnut mixture to coat on both sides. Place the coated salmon on the baking sheet.

Bake for 7 minutes. Turn the salmon over, and bake for another 7 minutes, or to your desired doneness.

Serve with a sprinkle of broccoli sprouts.

□ □ □

ZUCCHINI PASTA WITH BROCCOLI SPROUTS PESTO

Total time: 20 minutes • Makes 4 servings

4 zucchinis	½ teaspoon sea salt
1 cup fresh basil	½ cup spinach
½ cup broccoli sprouts	2 cups raw walnuts
Juice of 1 lemon	½ cup extra-virgin olive oil (or more for smoother mixture)
4 garlic cloves	

Make thin strips of zucchini using a vegetable peeler or pasta machine. Set aside.

Place the remaining ingredients in a blender and blend until the pesto mixture reaches desired consistency. Add more olive oil, as desired. Set aside.

Distribute the zucchini evenly among 4 plates.

Pour the pesto sauce over the zucchini pasta and serve.

□ □ □

MASHED CAULIFLOWER

Total time: 15 minutes • Makes 4 servings

1 head of cauliflower, cut into bite-size pieces	Sea salt and pepper, to taste
1 tablespoon olive oil or coconut oil	

Bring a large pot of water to boil. Add the cauliflower and cook until very tender, about 10 minutes.

Drain the water, then transfer the cauliflower to a food processor. Add the oil, sea salt, and pepper and process until smooth. (You could also mash the cauliflower by hand the traditional way, but a food processor will make sure the mash is extremely creamy.)

Add filtered water, more oil, or almond milk, until you reach the desired consistency.

TIP: Replace half the cauliflower with 1 to 2 white potatoes for Potato-Cauliflower Mash.

□ □ □

BONE BROTH

Total time: 30 minutes prep, 24 hours cooking • Makes 9 cups

Bones from 2 chickens (approx. 2½ pounds of chicken bones) or 2½ pounds of grass-fed beef bones

2 tablespoons apple cider vinegar

1 teaspoon sea salt

1 teaspoon turmeric

½ teaspoon black pepper

½ inch ginger root, peeled and chopped

1 medium onion, peeled and quartered

½ head of broccoli, chopped into chunks

2 celery stalks, cut into thirds

2 carrots, peeled and halved

2 garlic cloves, smashed

1 bay leaf

2 rosemary sprigs

1 tablespoon dried oregano or oregano essential oil

20 cups filtered water

Add all the ingredients to a large pot and bring to a boil. Once the liquid is boiling vigorously, lower the heat, cover, and simmer for 24 hours.

Check the broth every few hours and stir. You will know it's cooked when you poke the bones with a fork and they fall apart and break.

When the broth is done, strain it through mesh so you are left with just the liquid. Discard the solids.

TIPS:

- You can also put the ingredients into a slow cooker and let the broth cook for 8 to 12 hours.

- Some people like to roast their chicken bones before boiling them for a smoky flavor. You can also buy two organic rotisserie chickens instead of roasting your own.

- If you store bone broth in the fridge, it will set hard, which is a good sign that the marrow nutrients came out of the bones. It will become liquid again once heated.

- Store in the fridge for up to 6 days or in the freezer for up to 4 months. If freezing, allow extra room in the container, as it will expand when frozen.

RECOMMENDED RESOURCES

Videos

The Mysterious World under the Skin
A fascinating 42-minute documentary, free on YouTube, that explores state-of-the-art fascia research.

Fascia Research Congress
Enter the search term "Fascia Research Congress" in YouTube, and you'll discover a wealth of free videos by leading researchers in the fascia movement.

Books

Fascial Fitness: How to Be Vital, Elastic, and Dynamic in Everyday Life and Sport, by Robert Schleip (with Johanna Bayer), Lotus Publishing, 2017
A fun, easy-to-read book by one of the leading researchers in the fascia community.

Fascia in Sport and Movement, edited by Robert Schleip, Handspring Publishing, 2015
An outstanding guide for athletes, coaches, trainers, and therapists.

Anatomy Trains, by Thomas W. Myers, Churchill Livingston, 2014
An excellent resource for professionals who want an in-depth look into the anatomy and physiology of the fascia.

Fascia: What It Is and Why It Matters, by David Lesondak, Handspring Publishing, 2017

A good next step for both lay readers and professionals who want a deeper understanding of the fascia.

The MELT Method, by Sue Hitzmann, HarperOne, 2013
A step-by-step guide to Sue's method (for more on the MELT Method, see page 129).

Quench: Beat Fatigue, Drop Weight, and Heal Your Body through the New Science of Optimum Hydration, by Dana Cohen, M.D., and Gina Bria, Hatchette, 2018
An eye-opening look at why dehydration is epidemic and how it affects all areas of the body, including the fascia.

The Earth Diet (2014), *Cancer-Free with Food* (2019), and *10-Minute Recipes* (2016), by Liana Werner-Gray, Hay House
Three highly recommended resources for readers interested in optimizing their health—including the health of their fascia—by making smart food choices.

A Headache in the Pelvis, by David Wise and Rodney Anderson, M.D., Harmony, 2018
An absolute must-read if you are one of the millions of men and women suffering from unexplained pain in the pelvic region.

Websites

Jean-Claude Guimberteau, M.D.
www.guimberteau-jc-md.com/en/

Robert Schleip, Ph.D., Somatics
www.somatics.de/en/schleip

Tom Myers, Anatomy Trains
https://www.anatomytrains.com

Aaron Mattes, M.S., Stretching USA
https://www.stretchingusa.com

Alice Norton, MPH, low-oxalate diet
https://sallyknorton.com

Antonio Stecco, M.D., Hands on Seminars
https://www.handsonseminars.com/our_team/dr-antonio-stecco

Sabrina Atkins, D.C., Orlando Sports Chiropractic
www.orlandosportschiropractic.com/meet-dr-sabrina

Ida Rolf Institute
https://rolf.org

Environmental Working Group (EWG). (Check out their "Dirty Dozen" and "Clean Fifteen" lists, as well as the Skin Deep Database.)
https://www.ewg.org

Conference

The Fascia Research Congress meets regularly to disseminate the latest findings in the field. For information, see https://fascia congress.org.

ENDNOTES

Chapter 1

1. Petros C. Benias et al. "Structure and Distribution of an Unrecognized Interstitium in Human Tissues," *Scientific Reports*, 8, March 27, 2018, 4947, https://www.nature.com/articles/s41598-018-23062-6. See also: NYU Langone Health. "Newfound 'organ' had been missed by standard method for visualizing anatomy," Medical Xpress, March 27, 2018, https://medicalxpress.com/news/2018-03-newfound-standard-method-visualizing-anatomy.html.

2. As described by Dr. Wilke in the documentary *The Mysterious World under the Skin*, Dr. J.C. Guimberteau/EndoVivoProductions, produced by doc.station for ZDF in cooperation with Arte.

3. L. Berrueta et al. "Stretching Reduces Tumor Growth in a Mouse Breast Cancer Model," *Scientific Reports*, 8, May 18, 2018, 7864, https://doi.org/10.1038/s41598-018-26198-7.

4. Robert Schleip and Heike Jäger. "Interoception. A new correlate for intricate connections between fascial receptors, emotion and self recognition," from *Fascia—the Tensional Network of the Human Body*, R. Schleip, T. Findley, L. Chaitow, and P. Huijing, eds., Elsevier, 2012.

5. Zehra Gok Metin et al. "Aromatherapy Massage for Neuropathic Pain and Quality of Life in Diabetic Patients," *Journal of Nursing Scholarship*, 49(4), July 2017, 379–88, https://doi.org/10.1111/jnu.12300.
   Sudarshan Anandkumar et al. "Effect of fascia dry needling on non-specific thoracic pain—a proposed dry needling grading system," *Physiotherapy Theory and Practice*, 33(5), 2017, https://doi.org/10.1080/09593985.2017.1318423.
   Sannasi Rajasekar and Aurélie Marie Marchand. "Fascial Manipulation® for persistent knee pain following ACL and meniscus repair," *Journal of Bodywork and Movement Therapies*, 21(2), April 2017, 452–58, https://doi.org/10.1016/j.jbmt.2016.08.014.
   Sivan Navot and Leonid Kalichman. "Hip and groin pain in a cyclist resolved after performing a pelvic floor fascial mobilization," *Journal of Bodywork and Movement Therapies*, 20(3), July 2016, 604–9, https://doi.org/10.1016/j.jbmt.2016.04.005.
   Danuta Lietz-Kijak et al. "Assessment of the Short-Term Effectiveness of Kinesiotaping and Trigger Points Release Used in Functional Disorders of the Masticatory Muscles," *Pain Research and Management*, May 10, 2018, 5464985, https://doi.org/10.1155/2018/5464985.
   Ali Ghanbari et al. "Migraine responds better to a combination of medical therapy and trigger point management than routine medical therapy alone," *NeuroRehabilitation*, 37(1), 2015, 157–63, https://doi.org/10.3233/NRE-151248.

Marco Pintucci et al. "Evaluation of fascial manipulation in carpal tunnel syndrome: a pilot randomized clinical trial," *European Journal of Physical and Rehabilitation Medicine*, 53(4), August 2017, 630–31, https://doi.org/10.23736/S1973-9087.17.04732-3.

6. I-Chen Liao et al. "Effects of Massage on Blood Pressure in Patients with Hypertension and Prehypertension: A Meta-analysis of Randomized Controlled Trials," *Journal of Cardiovascular Nursing*, 31(1), January–February 2016, 73–83, https://doi.org/10.1097/JCN.0000000000000217.

7. M. Shah et al. "Neuromuscular taping reduces blood pressure in systemic arterial hypertension," *Medical Hypotheses*, 116, July 2018, 30–32, https://doi.org/10.1016/j.mehy.2018.04.014.

8. Majid Emtiazy and Mahboobeh Abrishamkar. "The Effect of Massage Therapy on Children's Learning Process: A Review," *Iranian Journal of Medical Sciences*, 41(3 Suppl), May 2016, S64, https://www.ncbi.nlm.nih.gov/pubmed/27840530.
    H. Tang et al. "Treatment of insomnia with shujing massage therapy: a randomized controlled trial" [in Chinese], *Zhongguo Zhen Jiu*, 35(8), August 2015, 816–18, https://www.ncbi.nlm.nih.gov/pubmed/26571900.
    Samaneh Mansouri et al. "A placebo-controlled clinical trial to evaluate the effectiveness of massaging on infantile colic using a random-effects joint model," *Pediatric Health, Medicine and Therapeutics*, 9, November 16, 2018, 157–63, https://doi.org/10.2147/PHMT.S185214.

9. Maria Hernandez-Reif et al. "Premenstrual symptoms are relieved by massage therapy," *Journal of Psychosomatic Obstetrics & Gynecology*, 21(1), April 2000, 9–15, https://doi.org/10.3109/01674820009075603.

10. Tiffany Field et al. "Labor pain is reduced by massage therapy," *Journal of Psychosomatic Obstetrics & Gynecology*, 18(4), 1997, https://doi.org/10.3109/01674829709080701.

11. Tiffany Field. "Pregnancy and labor massage," *Expert Review of Obstetrics & Gynecology*, 5(2), March 2010, 177–81, https://doi.org/10.1586/eog.10.12.

12. Jerome M. Weiss. "Pelvic floor myofascial trigger points: manual therapy for interstitial cystitis and the urgency-frequency syndrome," *The Journal of Urology*, 166(6), December 2001, 2226–31, https://doi.org/10.1016/S0022-5347(05)65539-5.

13. I. Martínez-Hurtado et al. "Effects of diaphragmatic myofascial release in gastroesophageal reflux disease: a preliminary randomized controlled trial," *Scientific Reports*, 9, May 13, 2019, 7273, https://doi.org/10.1136/bmj.c332.

14. Tugba Aydin et al. "The Effectiveness of Dry Needling and Exercise Therapy in Patients with Dizziness Caused by Cervical Myofascial Pain Syndrome; Prospective Randomized Clinical Study," *Pain Medicine*, 20(1), January 2019, 153–60, https://doi.org/10.1093/pm/pny072.

15. Vilma Ćosić et al. "Fascial Manipulation® method applied to pubescent postural hyperkyphosis: a pilot study," *Journal of Bodywork and Movement Therapies*, 18(4), October 2014, 608–15, https://doi.org/10.1016/j.jbmt.2013.12.011.
    Sunghak Byun and Dongwook Han. "The effect of chiropractic techniques on the Cobb angle in idiopathic scoliosis arising in adolescence," *Journal of Physical Therapy Science*, 28(4), April 2016, 1106–10, https://doi.org/10.1589/jpts.28.1106.

16. Budiman Minasny. "Understanding the Process of Fascial Unwinding," *International Journal of Therapeutic Massage & Bodywork*, 2(3), 2009, 10–17, https://doi.org/10.3822/ijtmb.v2i3.43. See also: Antonio Manuel Fernández-Pérez et al. "Effects of Myofascial Induction Techniques on Physiologic and Psychologic Parameters: A Randomized Controlled Trial," *The Journal of Alternative and Complementary Medicine*, 14(7), September 21, 2008, https://doi.org/10.1089/acm.2008.0117.

17. C. Fede et al. "Expression of the endocannabinoid receptors in human fascial tissue." *European Journal of Histochemistry*, 60(2643), April 11, 2016, 130–34, https://doi.org/10.4081/ejh.2016.2643. See also: "Expression of the endocannabinoid receptors in human fascial tissue," Fascia & Fitness, October 28, 2017, http://www.fascialfitness.net.au/articles/expression-of-the-endocannabinoid-receptors-in-human-fascial-tissue-2.

18. John M. McPartland et al. "Cannabimimetic Effects of Osteopathic Manipulative Treatment," *The Journal of the American Osteopathic Association*, 105(6), 283–91, June 2005, https://jaoa.org/article.aspx?articleid=2093088.

19. Hugh MacPherson et al. "Acupuncture and Counselling for Depression in Primary Care: A Randomized Controlled Trial," *PLOS Medicine*, 10(9), September 24, 2013, https://doi.org/10.1371/journal.pmed.1001518. See also: Andrew M. Seaman. "Acupuncture as good as counseling for depression: study," *Reuters*, September 24, 2013, https://www.reuters.com/article/us-acupuncture-depression/acupuncture-as-good-as-counseling-for-depression-study-idUSBRE98N17420130924.

Chapter 2

1. Tero A. H. Järvinen et al. "Organization and distribution of intramuscular connective tissue in normal and immobilized skeletal muscles. An immunohistochemical, polarization and scanning electron microscopic study," *Journal of Muscle Research and Cell Motility*, 23(3), 245–54, February 2002, https://doi.org/10.1023/A:1020904518336.

2. D. G. Lee et al. "Stability, continence and breathing: the role of fascia following pregnancy and delivery," *Journal of Bodywork and Movement Therapies*, 12(4), October 2008, 333–48, https://doi.org/10.1016/j.jbmt.2008.05.003.

3. Kenneth Hansraj. "Assessment of Stresses about the Cervical Spine: Caused by Posture and Position of the Head," New York Spine Surgery, 2014.

4. Laura Sullivan. "Keep Your Head Up: 'Text Neck' Takes a Toll on the Spine," The Two-Way (blog), NPR, November 20, 2014, https://www.npr.org/sections/thetwo-way/2014/11/20/365473750/keep-your-head-up-text-neck-can-take-a-toll-on-the-spine.

5. "Chronic Dehydration More Common Than You Think," CBS Miami online, July 2, 2013, https://miami.cbslocal.com/2013/07/02/chronic-dehydration-more-common-than-you-think.

6. Tammy Chang et al. "Inadequate Hydration, BMI, and Obesity among US Adults: NHANES 2009–2012." *Annals of Family Medicine*, 14(4), July/August 2016, 320–24, http://www.annfammed.org/content/14/4/320.full.

7. "Conclusions," *BioInitiative 2012: A Rationale for Biologically-based Exposure Standards for Low-Intensity Electromagnetic Radiation* (updated 2017), https://bioinitiative .org/conclusions.

8. Yufei Li et al. "Advanced Glycation End-Products Diminish Tendon Collagen Fiber Sliding," *Matrix Biology*, 32(3–4), January 2013, https://doi.org/10.1016 /j.matbio.2013.01.003.

9. Cleveland Clinic. "Why Smoking Will Worsen Your Chronic Pain," healthessentials, August 23, 2017, https://health.clevelandclinic.org/why-smoking-will -worsen-your-chronic-pain.
   American Academy of Orthopaedic Surgeons. "Surgery and Smoking," OrthoInfo, https://orthoinfo.aaos.org/en/treatment/surgery-and-smoking.

10. Antonio Stecco et al. "Fascial entrapment neuropathy," *Clinical Anatomy*, 32(7), October 2019, 883–90, https://doi.org/10.1002/ca.23388.

11. Simone Brandolini et al. "Sport injury prevention in individuals with chronic ankle instability: Fascial Manipulation® versus control group: a randomized controlled trial," *Journal of Bodywork and Movement Therapies*, 23(2), April 2019, 316–23, https://doi.org/10.1016/j.jbmt.2019.01.001.

Chapter 4

1. American Academy of Orthopaedic Surgeons, "Plantar fasciitis? Stretching seems to do the trick," ScienceDaily, November 4, 2010, https://www.sciencedaily .com/releases/2010/11/101104101657.htm.

2. Punjama Tunwattanapong et al. "The effectiveness of a neck and shoulder stretching exercise program among office workers with neck pain: a randomized controlled trial," *Clinical Rehabilitation*, March 16, 2015 (online), https:// doi.org/10.1177/0269215515575747.

3. Giwon Kim et al. "Effect of stretching-based rehabilitation on pain, flexibility and muscle strength in dancers with hamstring injury: a single-blind, prospective, randomized clinical trial," *Journal of Sports Medicine and Physical Fitness*, 58(9), September 2018, 1287–95, https://doi.org/10.23736/S0022 -4707.17.07554-5.
   Dayana P. Rosa et al. "Effects of a stretching protocol for the pectoralis minor on muscle length, function, and scapular kinematics in individuals with and without shoulder pain," *Journal of Hand Therapy*, 30(1), January–March 2017, 20–29, https://doi.org/10.1016/j.jht.2016.06.006.
   Ji-Eun Kim et al. "The effect of a Janda-based stretching program on range of motion, muscular strength, and pain in middle-aged women with self-reported muscular skeletal symptoms," *Journal of Exercise Rehabilitation*, 15(1), February 25, 2019, 123–28, https://doi.org/10.12965/jer.1836606.303.
   Mohammad Ghasemi et al. "The impacts of rest breaks and stretching exercises on lower back pain among commercial truck drivers in Iran," *International Journal of Occupational Safety and Ergonomics*, June 2018, 1–8, https://doi.org/10.1080/10803548.2018.1459093.

4. Jeffrey Gergley. "Acute Effect of Passive Static Stretching on Lower-Body Strength in Moderately Trained Men," *Journal of Strength and Conditioning Research*, 27(4), April 2013, 973–77, https://doi.org/10.1519/JSC.0b013e318260b7ce.

5. L. Berrueta et al. "Stretching Reduces Tumor Growth in a Mouse Breast Cancer Model," *Scientific Reports*, 8, May 18, 2018, 7864, https://www.nature.com /articles/s41598-018-26198-7. See also: Brigham and Women's Hospital. "Downward-facing mouse: stretching reduces tumor growth in mouse model of breast cancer," Medical XPress, May 22, 2018, https://medicalxpress.com /news/2018-05-downward-facing-mouse-tumor-growth-breast.html.

Chapter 5

1. Erik Peper and I-Mei Lin. "Increase or Decrease Depression: How Body Postures Influence Your Energy Level," *Biofeedback*, 40(3), Fall 2012, 125–30, https:// doi.org/10.5298/1081-5937-40.3.01.

2. Hamayun Zafar et al. "Effect of Different Head-Neck Postures on the Respiratory Function in Healthy Males," *BioMed Research International*, July 12, 2018, 4518269, https://doi.org/10.1155/2018/4518269.

3. Shwetha Nair et al. "Do slumped and upright postures affect stress responses? A randomized trial," *Health Psychology*, 34(6), June 2015, 632–41, https://doi.org /10.1037/hea0000146.

Chapter 6

1. Yuan-Chi Chan et al. "Short-term effects of self-massage combined with home exercise on pain, daily activity, and autonomic function in patients with myofascial pain dysfunction syndrome," *Journal of Physical Therapy Science*, 27(1), January 2015, 217–21, https://doi.org/10.1589/jpts.27.217.

2. A. R. Mohr et al. "Effect of foam rolling and static stretching on passive hip-flexion range of motion," *Journal of Sport Rehabilitation*, 23(4), November 2014, 296–99, https://doi.org/10.1123/jsr.2013-0025.

3. Lewis J. Macgregor et al. "The Effect of Foam Rolling for Three Consecutive Days on Muscular Efficiency and Range of Motion," *Sports Medicine—Open*, 4(26), 2018, https://sportsmedicine-open.springeropen.com/articles/10.1186/s40798 -018-0141-4. See also: "Foam rolling warm-up enhances performance," University of Stirling, June 15, 2018, https://www.stir.ac.uk/news/2018/06/foam -rolling-warm-up-enhances-performance.

4. Gregory E. P. Pearcey et al. "Foam Rolling for Delayed-Onset Muscle Soreness and Recovery of Dynamic Performance Measures," *Journal of Athletic Training*, 50(1), January 2015, 5–13, https://doi.org/10.4085/1062-6050-50.1.01.

5. Takanobu Okamoto et al. "Acute Effects of Self-Myofascial Release Using a Foam Roller on Arterial Function," *Journal of Strength and Conditioning Research*, 28(1), January 2014, 69–73, https://doi.org/10.1519/JSC.0b013e31829480f5.

6. Jan Wilke et al. "Immediate effects of self-myofascial release on latent trigger point sensitivity: a randomized, placebo-controlled trial," *Biology of Sport*, 35(4), December 2018, 349–54, https://doi.org/10.5114/biolsport.2018.78055.

7. Scott W. Cheatham. "Roller Massage: A Descriptive Survey of Allied Health Professionals," *Journal of Sport Rehabilitation*, 28(6), October 28, 2018, 640–49, https://doi.org/10.1123/jsr.2017-0366.

8. Benjamin S. Killen et al. "Crossover Effects of Unilateral Static Stretching and Foam Rolling on Contralateral Hamstring Flexibility and Strength," *Journal of Sport Rehabilitation*, 28(6), 2019, 533–39, https://doi.org/10.1123/jsr.2017-0356.

Chapter 7

1. Yufei Li et al. "Advanced Glycation End-Products Diminish Tendon Collagen Fiber Sliding," *Matrix Biology*, 32(3–4), January 2013, https://doi.org/10.1016/j.matbio.2013.01.003.

2. Chetan Sharma et al. "Advanced glycation end-products (AGEs): an emerging concern for processed food industries," *Journal of Food Science and Technology*, 52(12), December 2015, 7561–76, https://link.springer.com/article/10.1007/s13197-015-1851-y.

3. Tamsyn S. A. Thring et al. "Anti-collagenase, anti-elastase and anti-oxidant activities of extracts from 21 plants," *BMC Complementary and Alternative Medicine*, 9(27), 2009, https://doi.org/10.1186/1472-6882-9-27. See also: Kingston University. "White Tea Could Keep You Healthy and Looking Young," ScienceDaily, August 14, 2009, https://www.sciencedaily.com/releases/2009/08/090810085312.htm.

4. D. Sharan et al. "Effect of yoga on the Myofascial Pain Syndrome of neck," *International Journal of Yoga*, 7(1), January–June 2014, 54–59, https://doi.org/10.4103/0973-6131.123486.

5. Daniel J. DeNoon. "Tai Chi: Best Fibromyalgia Treatment? Study Shows Fibromyalgia Symptoms Much Better after 12 Weeks of Tai Chi," WebMD, August 18, 2010, https://www.webmd.com/fibromyalgia/news/20100818/tai-chi-best-fibromyalgia-treatment#1.

6. Vicki Contie. "Yoga or Stretching Eases Low Back Pain," NIH Research Matters, October 31, 2011, https://www.nih.gov/news-events/nih-research-matters/yoga-or-stretching-eases-low-back-pain.

7. Robert B. Saper et al. "Yoga, Physical Therapy, or Education for Chronic Low Back Pain: A Randomized Noninferiority Trial," *Annals of Internal Medicine*, 167(2), July 18, 2017, 85–94, https://doi.org/10.7326/M16-2579.

8. Arrate Pinto-Carral et al. "Pilates for women with breast cancer: a systematic review and meta-analysis," *Complementary Therapies in Medicine*, 41, December 2018, 130–40, https://doi.org/10.1016/j.ctim.2018.09.011.

9. Lynne Gaskell and Anita E. Williams. "A qualitative study of the experiences and perceptions of adults with chronic musculoskeletal conditions following a 12-week Pilates exercise programme," *Musculoskeletal Care*, 17(1), March 2019, 54–62, https://doi.org/10.1002/msc.1365.

10. Rafael Lomas-Vega et al. "Tai Chi for Risk of Falls. A Meta-analysis," *Journal of the American Geriatrics Society*, 65(9), September 2017, 2037–43, https://doi.org/10.1111/jgs.15008.

11. Judith T. Moskowitz et al. "Randomized controlled trial of a facilitated online positive emotion regulation intervention for dementia caregivers," *Health Psychology*, 38(5), May 2019, 391–402, https://psycnet.apa.org/record/2019-23038-008. See also: Allison Aubrey. "From Gloom to Gratitude: 8 Skills to Cultivate

Joy," Shots: Health News from NPR, NPR, May 5, 2019, https://www.npr.org /sections/health-shots/2019/05/05/719780061/from-gloom-to-gratitude-8 -skills-to-cultivate-joy.

12. Louise Hay, *I Can Do It: How to Use Affirmations to Change Your Life*. Carlsbad, CA: Hay House, 2004.

13. Christopher N. Cascio et al. "Self-affirmation activates brain systems associated with self-related processing and reward and is reinforced by future orientation," *Social Cognitive and Affective Neuroscience*, 11(4), April 2016, 621–29, https://doi.org/10.1093/scan/nsv136.

Chapter 8

1. Cited in "What Research Shows about Chiropractic," American Chiropractic Association, https://www.acatoday.org/Patients/Why-Choose-Chiropractic /What-Research-Shows.

2. Benjamin J. Keeney et al. "Early Predictors of Lumbar Spine Surgery after Occupational Back Injury: Results from a Prospective Study of Workers in Washington State," *Spine*, 38(11), May 15, 2013, 953–64, https://doi.org/10.1097 /BRS.0b013e3182814ed5.

3. James M. Whedon et al. "Association between Utilization of Chiropractic Services for Treatment of Low-Back Pain and Use of Prescription Opioids," *The Journal of Alternative and Complementary Medicine*, 24(6), June 2018, https://doi .org/10.1089/acm.2017.0131.

4. Cynthia English and Elizabeth Keating. "Majority in U.S. Say Chiropractic Works for Neck, Back Pain," Well-Being, Gallup, September 8, 2015, https:// news.gallup.com/poll/184910/majority-say-chiropractic-works-neck-back-pain .aspx.

5. Robert Granter. *The Myofascial Vacuum Cupping Manual*, Australasian College of Soft Tissue Therapy, 2010, PDF.

6. D. Murray and C. Clarkson. "Effects of moving cupping therapy on hip and knee range of movement and knee flexion power: a preliminary investigation," *Journal of Manual and Manipulative Therapy*, 27(5), December 2019, 287–94, https://doi.org/10.1080/10669817.2019.1600892.

7. Alycia Markowski et al. "A Pilot Study Analyzing the Effects of Chinese Cupping as an Adjunct Treatment for Patients with Subacute Low Back Pain on Relieving Pain, Improving Range of Motion, and Improving Function," *The Journal of Alternative and Complementary Medicine*, 20(2), December 2013, https://doi .org/10.1089/acm.2012.0769.

8. Shirin Mohammadi et al. "The effects of cupping therapy as a new approach in the physiotherapeutic management of carpal tunnel syndrome," *Physiotherapy Research International*, 24(3), July 2019, e1770, https://doi.org/10.1002/pri.1770.

9. Seoyoun Kim et al. "Is cupping therapy effective in patients with neck pain? A systematic review and meta-analysis," *BMJ Open*, 8(11), November 5, 2018, e021070, https://doi.org/10.1136/bmjopen-2017-021070.

10. Helene M. Langevin. "The Science of Stretch," *The Scientist*, May 1, 2013, https://www.the-scientist.com/features/the-science-of-stretch-39407.

11. Jennifer A. M. Stone and Peter A. S. Johnstone. "Mechanisms of Action for Acupuncture in the Oncology Setting," *Current Treatment Options in Oncology*, 11(3–4), December 2010, 118–27, https://doi.org/10.1007/s11864-010-0128-y.

12. "Acupuncture: In Depth," National Center for Complementary and Integrative Health, updated January 2016, https://nccih.nih.gov/health/acupuncture/introduction.

13. Tiffany Field. "Massage therapy research review," *Complementary Therapies in Clinical Practice*, 20(4), November 2014, 224–29, https://doi.org/10.1016/j.ctcp.2014.07.002.

14. Ibid.

15. Daniel C. Cherkin et al. "A Comparison of the Effects of 2 Types of Massage and Usual Care on Chronic Low Back Pain: A Randomized, Controlled Trial," *Annals of Internal Medicine*, 155(1), July 5, 2011, 1–9, https://doi.org/10.7326/0003-4819-155-1-201107050-00002.

16. Simone S. M. Ho et al. "Experiences of aromatherapy massage among adult female cancer patients: a qualitative study," *Journal of Clinical Nursing*, 26(23–24), December 2017, 4519–26, https://doi.org/10.1111/jocn.13784.

17. Tiffany Field et al. "Hand pain is reduced by massage therapy," *Complementary Therapies in Clinical Practice*, 17(4), November 2011, 226–29, https://doi.org/10.1016/j.ctcp.2011.02.006.

18. Justin D. Crane et al. "Massage Therapy Attenuates Inflammatory Signaling after Exercise-Induced Muscle Damage," *Science Translational Medicine*, 4(119), February 1, 2012, https://doi.org/10.1126/scitranslmed.3002882.

19. Yoon Soo Cho et al. "The effect of burn rehabilitation massage therapy on hypertrophic scar after burn: a randomized controlled trial," *Burns*, 40(8), December 2014, 1513–20, https://doi.org/10.1016/j.burns.2014.02.005.

20. Deborah Backus et al. "Impact of Massage Therapy on Fatigue, Pain, and Spasticity in People with Multiple Sclerosis: A Pilot Study," *International Journal of Therapeutic Massage and Bodywork*, 9(4), December 2016, 4–13, https://doi.org/10.3822/ijtmb.v9i4.327.

21. Seyhmus Kaplan et al. "Short-Term Effects of Kinesio Taping in Women with Pregnancy-Related Low Back Pain: A Randomized Controlled Clinical Trial," *Medical Science Monitor*, (22), April 18, 2016, 1297–1301, https://doi.org/10.12659/msm.898353.

22. Shu-Mei Chen et al. "Effects of Functional Fascial Taping on pain and function in patients with non-specific low back pain: a pilot randomized controlled trial," *Clinical Rehabilitation*, 26(10), October 2012, 924–33, https://doi.org/10.1177/0269215512441484.

23. I. Vithoulk et al. "The Effects of Kinesio Taping on Quadriceps Strength during Isokinetic Exercise in Healthy Non-athlete Women," *Isokinetics and Exercise Science*, 18(1), November 2009, https://doi.org/10.3233/IES-2010-0352.

24. Thiago Vilela Lemos et al. "The effect of Kinesio Taping on handgrip strength," *Journal of Physical Therapy Science*, 27(3), March 2015, 567–70, https://doi.org /10.1589/jpts.27.567.

25. Banu Ordahan et al. "Extracorporeal Shockwave Therapy versus Kinesiology Taping in the Management of Plantar Fasciitis: A Randomized Clinical Trial," *Archives of Rheumatology*, 32(3), September 2017, 227–33, https://doi.org /10.5606/ArchRheumatol.2017.6059.

26. Sayed A. Tantawy et al. "Comparative Study Between the Effects of Kinesio Taping and Pressure Garment on Secondary Upper Extremity Lymphedema and Quality of Life following Mastectomy: A Randomized Controlled Trial," *Integrative Cancer Therapies*, 18, May 8, 2019, 1534735419847276, https://doi .org/10.1177/1534735419847276.

27. Nihan Karatas et al. "The Effect of KinesioTape Application on Functional Performance in Surgeons Who have Musculo-skeletal Pain after Performing Surgery," *Turkish Neurosurgery*, 22(1), 2012, 83–89.

28. Leonid Kalichman and Simon Vulfsons. "Dry Needling in the Management of Musculoskeletal Pain," *Journal of the American Board of Family Medicine*, 23(5), September–October 2010, 640–46, https://doi.org/10.3122/jabfm.2010.05.090296.

29. Ibid.

30. Peter T. Dorsher and J. Fleckenstein. "Trigger Points and Classical Acupuncture Points," *Deutsche Zeitschrift für Akupunktur*, 51(4), October 2008, 6–11, https:// link.springer.com/article/10.1016/j.dza.2008.10.001. See also: "Mayo Clinic study shows acupuncture and myofascial trigger therapy treat same pain areas," Medical Xpress, May 13, 2008, https://medicalxpress.com/news/2008 -05-mayo-clinic-acupuncture-myofascial-trigger.html.

31. Harvey W. Wallmann et al. "The effects of whole body vibration on vertical jump, power, balance, and agility in untrained adults," *The International Journal of Sports Physical Therapy*, 14(1), February 2019, 55–64, https://www.ncbi .nlm.nih.gov/pmc/articles/PMC6350657.
    Atefeh Aminian-Far et al. "Whole-Body Vibration and the Prevention and Treatment of Delayed-Onset Muscle Soreness," *Journal of Athletic Training*, 46(1), January–February 2011, 43–49, https://doi.org/10.4085/1062-6050-46.1.43.

INDEX

NOTE: Page references in *italics* refer to photos.

V

W

Y

Z

ACKNOWLEDGMENTS

While this book has my name on it, it's the product of many generous people who have informed, inspired, and supported me.

I would like to thank The Fascia Research Society for the outstanding work they are doing in advancing the understanding of the role of fascia in health and wellness. Additionally, I would like to thank all the members of the society who contributed their knowledge, expertise, and time to help make this book possible. In particular, I'm very grateful to Dr. Robert Schleip for introducing me to many of his colleagues around the world.

I would like to thank Dr. Sheila K. Laws, who first opened my eyes to the complexity of soft tissue. Thank you to all chiropractors who have been promoting the concept of the body as one whole integrated system since September 18, 1895—the date of the first chiropractic treatment.

In addition, I owe a debt of gratitude to the entire team at Complete Wellness NYC for their help, which included everything from contributing their professional insights and stories to posing for photos. A special thank-you goes to Liana Werner-Gray for her contribution of recipes and the foreword to this book—and, even more importantly, for her inspiration and leadership in my becoming an author.

I would like to thank Wanda Hughes, Avi Korman, and Rebekah Fenster for being such great models for the photos. Thank you to Shreya Biswal for contributing her skills as a photographer. Thanks are due as well to my agent, Margot Maley Hutchison, for believing in this book, and to my editor, Nicolette Salamanca Young, and the remarkable production team at Hay House for making it a reality. This book would not be possible without the guidance and help of Alison Blake—I am forever grateful.

And finally, my thanks to my wife, Jan, and my children for lending their help every step of the way.

ABOUT THE AUTHOR

Daniel Fenster, D.C., is Clinic Director and Lead Chiropractor of Complete Wellness NYC. He graduated from Life Chiropractic College in Marietta, Georgia, in 1984 and has been practicing in New York City since 1985.

Dr. Fenster created Complete Wellness in 2007 with the vision of treating patients with a unified, synergistic approach by merging essential services and highly skilled providers under one roof. Today, this integrated wellness center is staffed by top health-care professionals in acupuncture and cupping, chiropractic, corrective one-on-one yoga, medical massage, medical pain relief, platelet-rich plasma injections, physical therapy, regenerative medicine, whole-body cryotherapy, nutrition for weight loss and optimal health, and more.

Dr. Fenster's noninvasive and drugless philosophy of wellness and his commitment to treating the whole patient have made him the chiropractor of choice in New York and worldwide for business leaders, professionals, athletes, celebrities, authors and editors, and countless others. He has been flown around the world to treat members of royalty and VIPs.

Website: www.completewellnessnyc.com

We hope you enjoyed this Hay House book. If you'd like to receive our online catalog featuring additional information on Hay House books and products, or if you'd like to find out more about the Hay Foundation, please contact:

Hay House, Inc., P.O. Box 5100, Carlsbad, CA 92018-5100
(760) 431-7695 or (800) 654-5126
(760) 431-6948 (fax) or (800) 650-5115 (fax)
www.hayhouse.com® • www.hayfoundation.org

———

Published in Australia by: Hay House Australia Pty. Ltd.,
18/36 Ralph St., Alexandria NSW 2015
Phone: 612-9669-4299 • *Fax:* 612-9669-4144
www.hayhouse.com.au

Published in the United Kingdom by: Hay House UK, Ltd.,
The Sixth Floor, Watson House, 54 Baker Street, London W1U 7BU
Phone: +44 (0)20 3927 7290 • *Fax:* +44 (0)20 3927 7291
www.hayhouse.co.uk

Published in India by: Hay House Publishers India,
Muskaan Complex, Plot No. 3, B-2, Vasant Kunj, New Delhi 110 070
Phone: 91-11-4176-1620 • *Fax:* 91-11-4176-1630
www.hayhouse.co.in

———

Access New Knowledge.
Anytime. Anywhere.

Learn and evolve at your own pace
with the world's leading experts.

www.hayhouseU.com